BETTER VISION NOW
Improve Your Sight with the Renowned Bates Method

CLARA A. HACKETT

with LAWRENCE GALTON

Foreword by WILLIAM GUTMAN, M.D.

Illustrated by LAURA GLUSHA

DOVER PUBLICATIONS, INC.
Mineola, New York

Bibliographical Note

This Dover edition, first published in 2006, is an unabridged republication of
Relax and See: A Daily Guide to Better Vision, first published by Harper &
Brothers, New York, in 1955. The color plate originally appearing on page 77
has been reproduced in color on the inside front cover.

Library of Congress Cataloging-in-Publication Data

Hackett, Clara A.
   [Relax and see]
   Better vision now : improve your sight with the renowned Bates method /
Clara A Hackett, with Lawrence Galton.
      p. cm.
   Reprint. Originally published: Relax and see. New York : Harper, 1955.
   Includes index.
   ISBN-13: 978-0-486-45253-1 (pbk.)
   ISBN-10: 0-486-45253-0 (pbk.)
    1. Bates method of orthoptics. 2. Vision disorders—Alternative treatment.
3. Vision disorders—Prevention. I. Galton, Lawrence. II. Title.

RE992.O7H3 2006
617.7—dc22

                    2006046264

Manufactured in the United States by Courier Corporation
45253007   2014
www.doverpublications.com

Contents

Illustrations

I wish to pay tribute to the memory of my mother who always insisted that there would be a way to restore my sight.

I also wish to thank the persons who gave suggestions and time in preparing this book. They are:

Dorothy Clifford
Gertrude Donahue
Dorothy Cooke Federlein
Caroline Flanders
Waldo Glaser
Jean Hersey
Robert W. Hersey
Paul Hester, S.J.
S. Rutherford Olliphant
Jack Stites
Marie Strack
Marion Patton Waldron

Foreword

The principle of systematic exercise and training, generally applied in the treatment and rehabilitation of the crippled and handicapped, has been strangely enough more or less overlooked for a long time in the field of disturbances of the visual function.

It was Dr. Bates who introduced this general principle of treatment for the first time on a larger scale into ophthalmology. Since its first introduction, several books dealing with this method have been published. However, so far there has been no book which could serve as a definite and practical guide for the many who want to improve their vision through systematic eyesight training. Miss Hackett's book fills this gap admirably.

Through many innovations and a skillful blending of techniques, the author has created an easy-to-follow, step-by-step method to help to improve general poor seeing habits, to help to make the best possible use of remaining vision in severer disturbances and finally to improve even organic conditions through creating better function of the eye.

The modern functional and psychosomatic approach in medicine which recognizes and utilizes the influence of function upon structure and of mind upon the body finds its expression also in such methods as the one described in this book. Better function reduces strain, thus providing better nourishment of the organ and building of healthier tissue, leading to regeneration of pathological structure.

On the other hand, we know that we function as a perfect unit of mind and body, one influencing the other, and that we see not only with the eye, but also with the brain and the mind.

The methods described in *Relax and See* follow these modern concepts in medicine and lead through relaxation, training of the visual function and skillful use of psychological factors to better vision.

The proof of the pudding is in the eating. I have seen excellent results of this system of eyesight training in a great number of cases, even when severe pathology was present. Having become interested in it, I myself experienced improvement of vision through the application of Miss Hackett's method. It is hoped that now many more will be enabled to have the same experience.

WILLIAM GUTMAN, M.D.

Preface

This book is an attempt to put into the hands not of a select few but of the great majority of people who might benefit by it, a simple method of improving eyesight—clear, detailed and with the step-by-step, day-to-day procedure so well defined that it can be readily applied by any intelligent person.

It is now some thirty-five years since Dr. William H. Bates, a practicing New York City ophthalmologist, first demonstrated that visual training can bring marked improvement in eyesight. Since then, thousands of people have been helped by the methods devised by Dr. Bates and his pupils. But it is also true that help has been denied to the great majority of people with defective vision.

Not thousands, but millions—more than two-thirds of all adults in the United States, according to the Better Vision Institute—suffer from defective vision. The relatively few thousands who have benefited from vision re-education have been the fortunate people who could find well-trained teachers, of whom there are all too few. By and large, too, most of the beneficiaries have been people with urgent need —men and women to whom poor eyesight was an overwhelming handicap, an obstacle in careers where perfect or almost perfect vision is essential. They have been able and willing, indeed eager, because of the seriousness of their problem, to devote many hours a day, over long periods, sometimes at considerable expense, to improving sight.

No significant development ever springs into being fullblown, with all the tools and techniques needed to implement it effectively. Although the Bates theory of sight retraining is, in itself, simple, the problem has always been to find methods of putting it into practice most effectively. The need has been for techniques that not only produce better results for more people in faster time, but also for techniques that are simple to understand and easy to apply, that sustain interest and avoid boredom, that are practical for most people who haven't hours a day to devote to them and, let us be frank, who haven't the motivation to continue with drills that seem excessively demanding.

There has been a need, too, for a book which, in the absence of expert instruction, will permit people to make practical progress in improving their vision on their own.

It is the hope that the methods presented in this book and their way of presentation will help to fill both needs.

While many of the methods in the following chapters are those first used by Dr. Bates, there are also many new techniques based on original research.

During the last ten years I have worked with more than 2,800 people whose visual deficiencies ranged from nearsightedness and farsightedness to more serious problems such as glaucoma and cataracts.

Early in this work, it became apparent that modifications in established techniques could produce far better results. For example, open-eyed sunning, an early Bates procedure, has been most criticized by physicians as dangerous. A major purpose of sunning is to achieve eye relaxation—an essential step if there is to be an opportunity to displace bad visual habits. But open-eyed sunning for many people, even if not dangerous, is such an uncomfortable procedure that it defeats its purpose, for relaxation is hard to achieve in the presence of discomfort. I have found that taking light on closed lids not only accomplishes the same purpose without any possible danger but is even more effective because it can be done without discomfort.

The development of great variety in techniques has proved helpful. Many variations were suggested by students taking the training. The variety eliminates boredom.

After working with several hundred people, it became clear that, in virtually every sight disturbance, faulty fusion plays an important role which had not been recognized previously. Fusion is the combination of physical focusing and mental merging that causes the separate images from the two eyes to appear as one clear image in the brain. Even a slight deviation in fusion can cause a blurring of vision which, I suspect, accentuates or even brings on strain and faulty seeing habits and leads to progressive vision loss. Once the problem was recognized, methods of overcoming it were found. And fusion techniques have proved to be important in getting both faster and greater improvement in vision.

Most earlier systems of improving sight have limited themselves to black and white material. Encouraged by favorable results, I have employed color in many ways. Its use increases the interest in lessons. But, more than that, it is as necessary to restore the ability to see color as to see form. After all, we live in a world of color and not of eye charts!

Music, too, is emphasized and used almost continuously to make all activities rhythmical. Rhythm may be one of the deep secrets of life; perhaps, as Havelock Ellis has indicated in *The Dance of Life*, there are rhythm patterns of human behavior. I do not pretend to know how all-pervading rhythm is. My use of rhythm is empirical; I have found that it increases both the ease and the enjoyment of practice.

One of the most important developments of all, I believe, was the emphasis that came to be placed on casual practice —on making visual re-education not entirely a matter of formal drills in special periods set aside for them, but much more a matter of easy, inconspicuous, little, momentary diversions all day long and even an integrated part of regular activities. This accomplishes two purposes. The housewife, for example, who as part of overcoming her particular vision difficulty is told to watch the movement of her spoon as she stirs the pudding, has ready-made opportunity to practice. It is easier to spend more time in learning when the time does not have to be taken away from other activities. But, fully as important, the integration of good seeing practices into the whole fabric of daily life insures their continued automatic use as habits so that the improvement in vision will not be lost and continual routines or drills will not forever be necessary.

There is emphasis in this book, too, on measurement of progress. Not only does an awareness of progress lead to regularity and continuity of work that might otherwise be hard to achieve; it seems to be true, too, that the more a person thinks of himself as becoming normal-sighted, the more his sight improves because of the thinking. The mind, of course, is very much involved in seeing.

These methods have proved successful in 90 per cent of the 2,857 people I have personally instructed. They included 1,584 nearsighted persons, 348 farsighted, 248 bifocal wearers and 179 with squint or crossed-eye problems. There were also 312 with cataract, 35 with glaucoma, 55 with retinitis pigmentosa. Others included people with sight losses from retinitis and chorioretinitis, conical cornea, macular degeneration and atrophy of the optic nerve.

In addition to my own work, some sixty instructors whom I have trained have been able to help another 12,000 people. The methods presented in this book are now employed by members of the Hackett Eye Training Association who maintain offices in several states.

A few years ago, seventy nuns from Seattle's parochial schools took a brief course which I conducted at Seattle University. Their purpose was to apply selected techniques in the classrooms in an effort to prevent the development of eyesight defects in children. They have reported excellent results. In one classroom, for example, not a child has appeared in glasses since the techniques have been put into use. Incidentally, several other nuns in the Seattle parochial school system, who had been wearing glasses, became sufficiently impressed to decide to apply the techniques to themselves and were able to abandon glasses after a few months.

In writing this book I have had in mind the persons, far from a teacher, who have written letters to me that were pitiful. I have kept in mind the letter from an Indian woman whose mother, living on a reservation far from any city, had the diagnosis of cataract and a thirteen-year-old near-sighted girl who has written to me many times for help which was not available to her. In my files, too, are letters from thirty-seven states and nine foreign countries, from people as diverse in occupation as an engineer in Tunisia and a monk in the Middle West, all asking for help.

I have tried not only to set down the basic vision retraining techniques clearly but also to detail a definite program for their use in the solving of various types of vision problems. The explanation of principles and techniques is but the first part of effective teaching. It is equally important to guide the student in their use. The step-by-step plans in the later chapters of this book, which show the student exactly what he can do from day to day instead of leaving him with a list of techniques and the supplication to apply them somehow, are, I believe, a major strength of this book which will make it of practical value.

BETTER VISION NOW

Chapter I

The Case for Hope

Two of every three adults, many of them young, and a sizable proportion of children as well, today are limping along with defective eyesight. Seemingly, the only practical resort for them is to wear glasses.

No medical man, no eyesight specialist, claims that eyeglasses are more than a useful kind of crutch. They offer symptomatic relief, allowing more acute vision when worn. But they do not cure visual defects, do not touch causes.

Eyeglasses have their inconveniences, of course, producing a change in appearance not always considered desirable and sometimes imposing restraints on activity. They are annoying when they steam and fog, and when they break and have to be replaced.

But there is something much more disconcerting about them.

If you have defective vision and have worn glasses for some years, chances are you've had several changes of lens, each time to a stronger prescription. Your sight now, unaided by glasses, may not be nearly as good as it was when you first started wearing them. Your natural vision, it would seem, is becoming worse instead of better.

"Glasses," as Dr. Frank D. Costenbader, a distinguished ophthalmologist, recently reminded the National Society for the Prevention of Blindness, "only help the present but not the future of the wearer." They do nothing to halt progressive deterioration of sight. Indeed, there are those who believe that their very use contributes to deterioration.

1

Are glasses the only possible answer?

Are the eyes so different from all other body organs that, when they fail to function properly, there is no cure, no other help than a mechanical aid?

And are the eyes, to begin with, so inherently weak, and here again so different from all other body organs, that they should fail to such a huge extent—fail for at least two thirds of all persons and at such an early age?

Happily, the answer to all these questions is—no.

A CHECK FOR YOURSELF

In an ordinary business card, punch pinholes about ³⁄₁₆ of an inch apart so they make equilateral triangles, like this:

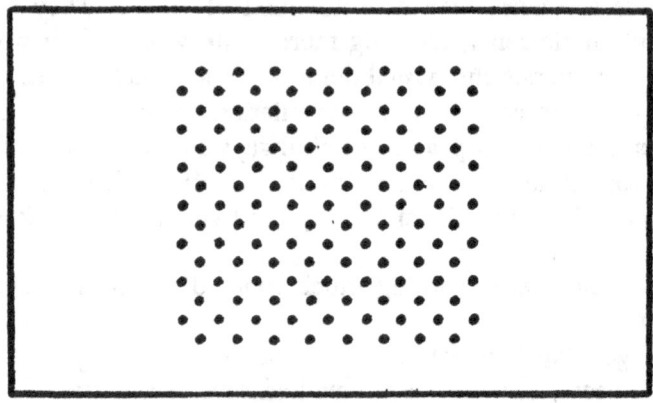

Fig. 1   Pinhole Check

Remove your glasses and look about you. You don't see well, of course. For this check, deliberately pick out a number of objects that you see as blurs. Make certain that all are in a good light.

Now, hold the card up before your eyes and look through the pinholes at the blurred objects. Don't stare. Don't try hard. Just glance at the objects casually.

If you do this properly, you'll be surprised to find that now, as you look through the pinholes on the card, there is a considerable improvement in your vision. The objects are no longer blurs. If your vision loss has not been severe, they may be quite sharp and clear. Even with severe vision impairment, they are far less hazy.

What you have just done is a happy demonstration, first, that you have greater potential vision, a greater natural power of sight than you may have dreamed. It also demonstrates, even if to only a limited extent, why you have lost good vision and how you can win it back. For, probably without realizing it, in order to see at all through the pinholes you had to use your sight in a different way, abandoning several poor vision habits in favor of proper ones. For example, you had to centralize instead of spread and blur your vision. Your sight, in shifting, was made extremely mobile. Centralization and mobility, as it will become clear later in this book, are just two of a number of vital habits that help to assure good vision.

It has long been a commonly accepted theory that when nearsightedness, farsightedness and other refractive errors occur, the trouble must lie in a defective lens or in other structural abnormalities of the eye. The solution has been to "correct for," or compensate for, the defect with glasses.

But there is another theory—and the pinhole check helps demonstrate it—that offers more hope. It holds that visual loss is not, invariably, the result of a fault in the lens or of a defect anywhere else in the structure of the eye. It proposes, instead, as we'll see in greater detail in Chapter II, that the trouble may be functional rather than organic. To put it another way, the eye itself may be perfect but use of it not; a major fault, and sometimes the only fault, may lie in poor visual habits, which were either learned originally or acquired later because of emotional problems or stress situations. As a natural corollary, this theory holds that correcting poor habits may stop further deterioration of already poor sight, and bring about correct rather than "corrected-for" vision.

How does this theory actually work out in practice? What can you expect to accomplish for your own sight if you are willing to do a few simple things each day?

If you have just tried the pinhole check, the improvement you noted represents your immediate potential sight—what your natural visual ability may be, unaided by glasses or by peering through pinholes, but looking about normally—in the near future, perhaps within six months or even less. Many people are able to double their sight—and some even triple it—within twelve weeks. The time required to achieve your immediate visual potential will depend not only on the amount of practice but on the extent of sight loss with which you start.

For example, if you are nearsighted, with a doctor's diagnosis of 20/40 vision now, your immediate potential may be 20/20—a doubling of your vision—and you may achieve it within twelve weeks. But if your sight now is only 20/400, one twentieth of normal vision, and your immediate potential is 20/50, in twelve weeks you may double your visual ability to 20/200, or even better, but it will take more months of practice before you can hope to achieve your immediate potential. Once you gain ground to this point, you may go on with further practice to achieve your ultimate potential of still greater, possibly even normal, vision.

For farsighted people, the outlook is the same. Suppose that, now, unaided by glasses, you can read, let us say, only the title of this book, but through the pinholes are able to read this print. Your immediate potential, which you are likely to achieve in a few months, will be the ability to read book print with your unaided eyes. At that point, you may be able to read, through the pinholes, the tiny print found in a later chapter, an indication of what your ultimate potential visual ability may be with further practice. These estimates are based on results achieved by almost 15,000 people with visual losses of various types who have retrained their vision under the supervision of myself and some sixty instructors. As I write this, I have before me the records of 2,857 with whom I worked personally.

The total figure of 2,857 includes some who had only a few lessons and stopped. It includes people who did not want to work for better sight—even those who did not want to see better. (If it seems impossible to imagine a person who does not want better sight, consider, as representative, an auto mechanic with such great vision loss that he has been classed as "occupationally blind" for ten years, and for whom regaining sight means loss of a pension and the need to return to work in a competitive field where he would have to learn newer skills. Although he may give lip service to the idea of trying to regain vision, he makes no real effort.)

My 2,857 students ranged in age from three to ninety-two years. Their occupations: machinists, stenographers, salesmen, lawyers, engineers, business executives, insurance agents, schoolteachers, ministers, housewives, accountants, priests, nuns, doctors and dentists.

There were 1,584 nearsighted people, or myopes, with vision ranging from 20/30 to 20/1000. The majority had 20/400, or one-twentieth of normal sight. Five hundred sixty-nine regained at least 20/40, or half normal sight; 210 achieved 20/70; 163 attained 20/100 or one-fifth normal sight; 211 improved to 20/200 or one-tenth of normal sight. In other cases there was lesser or only temporary improvement. All of those who achieved 20/20 vision could dispense with glasses as could most of those who gained 20/40, the sight required for passing drivers' tests in the states of New York, California and Washington. Most of the others had glasses prescribed for them that were from one to four diopters *weaker* than the pair being worn when they started their lessons.

Three hundred forty-eight of my students were farsighted; 116 discarded glasses entirely; 194 could wear weaker glasses for reading; 38 made no enduring improvement.

There were 248 bifocal wearers. Of these 84 discarded glasses entirely; 138 were able to substitute a light pair of reading glasses for their bifocals. The remaining 26 had no enduring benefit.

There were 179 cross-eyed students. Seventy-one have achieved straight eyes and also have good fusion; 96 have straight eyes and good fusion except that there is a slight deviation from the norm when they are ill, emotionally upset or fatigued. Twelve had no enduring improvement.

In all these cases, original diagnosis was made by physicians. Although it has been true that the medical profession has had reservations about the value of vision retraining, an increasing number of physicians in recent years have become impressed with the results. While some take the attitude: "It can do no harm," many others now believe it may do much good. Whether or not they express this publicly, they encourage many patients to try re-education.

I have had the privilege of working closely with many physicians more recently, not only in cases of refractive loss but also of serious eye disorders.

It must be emphasized that the vision retraining techniques presented in this book do not constitute a panacea. They are not intended to replace medical care. It is essential that people with actual diseases or growths in the eye seek medical aid. Self-diagnosis is never advisable. Only a physician is qualified to detect and identify disease.

In recent years, doctors who have encouraged patients with such serious disorders as glaucoma and cataracts to undertake vision retraining have found that astonishing improvement often occurs.

Thus far, I have worked with 312 people with cataracts. Of these, 278 had improvements ranging from 10 per cent better sight to complete normalcy, while only 34 had no noticeable lasting improvement. It is impossible to state how many had complete clearing of their cataracts for not all followed my request to return for medical re-examination; their increase of sight was proof enough for them that their cataracts were gone.

Forty of my recent students have had glaucoma. Of these, 11 gained greater field of vision and increased sight; 18 had a lowering of tension according to their doctors; 11 had no great lasting improvement, although 5 do report less pain and discomfort.

Fifty-seven persons with retinitis pigmentosa have had lessons. Of these, only 2 achieved 20/20 or normal sight; however, 38 had their field of vision and acuity helped appreciably even to the extent of driving a car again; 17 had no lasting benefit.

Of 31 persons with progressive sight losses from such diseases as retinitis, conical cornea, choreoretinitis, 10 have stopped the progression; they have been able to continue working at regular occupations, are no longer fearful of becoming incapacitated. One conical cornea case obtained 20/20 sight.

There have been worthwhile results in vision losses due to other serious problems and even in some blind people.

Blind persons must be classified according to whether they have only light perception, object perception, or more useful sight but are still considered "occupationally blind," or blind within the legal definition.

Of the 8 with only light perception who have had lessons, 1 is now working at his regular occupation, 4 others now have object perception. Three have had no improvement. Of 14 who had some object perception to begin with, 8 now have useful vision and are no longer "blindish." Six have had no lasting gain of sight. Of the 34 who had been considered occupationally blind, 16 are now working while 8 others have had increased sight. Ten have not improved appreciably.

No less important than improving vision defects is their prevention in the first place. Methods selected from those incorporated in this book are used in an eye-training program that many Seattle parochial schools have adopted. The program, under the direction of Dominican nuns who were trained by me at Seattle University, has shown its value in preserving and strengthening the sight of children.

HOW YOU WILL IMPROVE YOUR VISION

You will attain better vision not by long, complicated, vigorous exercises or by trying to bully your eyes into seeing better.

On the contrary, the whole emphasis will be on making vision effortless.

The very first step will be to achieve relaxation of the eyes. It is safe to say that you will find the relaxation techniques pleasurable. Moreover, they are likely to produce a highly desirable incidental benefit—relaxation throughout the body and in the mind. Relaxation not only will make your eyes feel rested but will provide the needed opening for establishing new habits.

To establish these habits, a certain number of drills will be necessary. They will be drills in fusion, in increasing mobility of sight, in producing centralized vision and in other proper habits of seeing. You will find them simple and easy to do. They are not exercises.

But a major emphasis will be on making the vision work a part of all your daily activities.

All of us, however busy, have almost limitless opportunities to integrate practice with our daily activities—if practice can be casual, if it can be easily and unobtrusively accomplished. You will find a great variety of techniques for such practice.

You will find that you will be able to practice better vision techniques in virtually every activity during the day —in walking, riding public conveyances, shaving, eating, watching movies and TV, playing cards, reading, writing, conversation, listening to music, dancing. The practice will not interfere with your enjoyment of these activities; in many, it will heighten it.

It is difficult to overcome bad habits and establish good ones unless one can be comfortable in the process. All of the techniques you will find in this book can be accomplished without discomfort. You need not be afraid that you must live entirely without glasses. You will go without them as much as you can—at first, for short periods only. Having used glasses for years, you cannot discard them at once. But as you progress, you will find it easy to dispense with them for increasingly long periods.

You will find your vision improving almost from day to day and you will be able to note your progress and to gain a great deal of encouragement from it.

You will not need to continue forever with the drills, except in retinitis pigmentosa and glaucoma. However, you may find that you will want to continue with a number of them because of the values they have outside of vision itself —in helping to relieve nervous tension and to heighten your awareness of the things going on around you, for example. Although you may have been using your eyes badly for twenty, thirty and even forty or fifty years, the techniques in this book, because they are so varied and can be used so effectively throughout the day instead of just in short formal periods of drilling, will establish new and proper habits of vision in a relatively short time. And, because of their all-day-long use, once such new habits have been established, the conscious techniques you have repeated over and over again day after day will be necessary no longer. The new habits will be just that—habits and almost entirely automatic.

HOW LONG WILL IT TAKE?

Defects in vision vary not only in kind but in degree. So does aptitude in following directions. So, too, motivation—

the depth of desire to achieve improvement which determines faithfulness in trying for it.

One of my students, a nearsighted young man (20/200), driven by a great desire to pass a Navy examination within a brief period of time, was able, by virtually giving up all other activity and concentrating on his eyesight, to bring his vision to 20/40 within a few weeks and pass the test. I have seen many other people with various types of vision deficiencies who, with sufficient desire, equaled this performance.

Most people, of course, progress in more leisurely fashion.

Another young man of twenty-five had had a crossed eye since childhood. He had undergone an operation on the eye solely for the purpose of getting a commission in the Navy. Despite the operation, however, the eye still deviated to such an extent, and the sight in it was so far below normal, that the Navy would not accept him. He still wanted his commission but there was no great urgency. It took six months before the cross was no longer noticeable and the vision was up to Navy standards.

A man in his fifties had worn reading glasses for twenty years and bifocals for one year. His sight for distance was normal within two months. Within a year, he was able to discard reading glasses entirely. He now reads two newspapers every day and at least three books a week—all without glasses.

A woman in her fifties with the doctor's diagnosis of cataracts in both eyes had 20/600 vision in one eye, 20/200 in the other. She had worn glasses for forty years and bifocals for twenty of them. In a year, her cataracts were gone, as attested by two physicians, and, now continuing her work in order to bring her sight up to normal, she has reached 20/30 in the better eye and 20/200 in the other. She can now read magazines and books entirely without glasses.

In cases of refractive error—in nearsightedness and farsightedness—with faithful work, it is often possible to double vision within twelve weeks. A farsighted person now able to read print, let us say, one-quarter of an inch high, may, within twelve weeks, be able to read print one-eighth of an inch high. A nearsighted person who now, at ten feet, can see a letter three inches high may be able, in the same length of time, to see a letter an inch and a half high at this distance.

Beyond this point, as in any other learning process, there is a slower rate of progress. In learning to type, for example, acquiring the fundamentals and a speed of, say, thirty words per minute may take less time than it requires to bring the speed up from thirty to sixty words per minute. Similarly, in retraining the vision, the first improvement is the fastest and the most dramatic. Thereafter, it may take four or five months to get the next doubling.

There is, of course, a natural human longing to know in advance what results can be expected and when. Fortunately, although this wish cannot be fully gratified, when it comes to vision retraining, this much can be said: There will be variations and some ups and down, but you will be able to know progress almost from the beginning.

THE EXTRA DIVIDENDS

Vision may influence the personality. Nearsighted people often tend to be shy and to suffer from a cruel inferiority complex. I have noted, as have their families and friends, how many women have bloomed and men taken on new stature after their handicap has been overcome.

Many farsighted people seem to be subject to great nervous tension which causes them to move too rapidly and to be somewhat diffuse in talking and perhaps even in thinking. Many have tremendous energy and sometimes use excessive amounts of it for unimportant purposes. As their sight improves, they report that they are physically and mentally more calm.

People who have been nearly blind, even when they have regained only a small part of their potential vision—when they reach the point where they can begin to engage in ordinary routine activities previously impossible, such as going to market—blossom forth with self-confidence that permeates their whole lives.

Another by-product of improved vision reported by many people is an improvement in memory. The nearsighted, for example, are often able to remember faces better; the far-sighted, the things they read.

Many nearsighted people gain a better ability to evaluate both space and motion. For example, when a nearsighted person who has had to wear glasses for driving brings his vision up to the point where he can pass a driving examination without the use of glasses, he finds that his depth perception has improved. He is able to park his car more easily.

One of the most important of all dividends that come from the improvement of vision is the loss of the fear of not being able to see properly on many occasions. Although we may not be aware of it, loss of vision does produce such a fear which often inhibits us. Nearsighted people, for example, commonly are afraid of, and avoid, looking off in the distance. Farsighted people are afraid to look in the telephone book for fear of not being able to read it. Some cross-eyed people are afraid to look other people in the face for fear that one more person in the world will know of their affliction. The cross-eyed person who avoids looking at people, the nearsighted one who avoids looking off in the distance, and the farsighted person who avoids looking at things at close hand miss a lot in life.

Other dividends have been noted, too, even during the course of establishing proper habits of vision. Ours is a tense civilization and the medical profession has shown an increasing tendency to trace many modern ills to tension. The techniques, developed over many years, for relaxation of the eyes are simple, practical, specific. A happy dividend of eye relaxation is relaxation elsewhere in the body. For the eyes are not set apart in the body. Many people who have suffered such ailments as migraine headaches and insomnia have discovered that they have had fewer headaches—in some cases, none at all—and far less trouble with sleeping after practicing eye relaxation.

WORKING WITH CHILDREN

The techniques given in this book have proved effective in improving vision in children as well as in adults. If you are an intelligent parent, disturbed over your child's visual handicap, the chances are great that you can help him to apply these techniques. A special chapter is devoted to specific suggestions for helping children.

It is fully as important to prevent loss of vision in children as it is to improve sight once loss has occurred. There are suggestions for this, too.

HOW TO USE THIS BOOK

It may seem presumptuous to tell you how to use a book. Yet these few suggestions may prove of value in saving time and effort for you. Your doctor has probably told you what your vision problem is. If not, you should ask for a diagnosis.

Whatever your particular problem, it is important for you to understand how the trouble developed. No attempt is made in this book to give you a detailed knowledge of the anatomy of the eye. But you will find in Chapter II a simple picture of the working of the eye and a discussion of how your particular problem may have developed, and this knowledge will buttress your efforts in retraining your vision.

Whatever your particular vision problem, a number of basic techniques apply to it as well as to all other vision problems. These techniques involve relaxation, fusion mobility, improving sight at all distances and the use of the mind in seeing. The reasons why these techniques are helpful in all types of vision problems will become clear as you follow the discussion about them in Chapters III to VII.

In Chapter VIII, you will find reading practice techniques that will be of value, and the two succeeding chapters are of vital importance because they show you how to use essential techniques in your daily life, in work and play.

I suggest, therefore, that you begin your work by carefully reading chapters I through X.

Thereafter, you will find one chapter which provides a step-by-step, week-by-week outline of the work to be done to overcome your problem. At the end of the book, you will also find a chapter on measuring your progress.

Chapter II

Why We Lose Sight

Although this is a wonderful era of technical accomplishment, no engineer could devise anything to equal the process by which you see. On a screen the size of a teaspoon bowl, the normal eye can pick up miles of landscape in the distance and a dot in a book—in life size and full color. Beyond the eye itself, with its exquisite construction, seeing also involves a precise and delicate mental performance. For we see *with* the eyes but *in* the brain, and the brain not only does the ultimate perceiving but also, without our conscious awareness regulates the eyes.

Considering the intricacy, it's a wonder vision does not fail completely more often than it does, that only about 250,000 of the 160,000,000 or more pairs of eyes in the country are blind. But it is not difficult to understand why imperfect vision, far short of blindness, is so common.

Although few of us realize it, seeing is an acquired skill. A newborn baby is almost blind and has to learn to see. Not all people learn any skill with equal facility. There are some who learn to walk gracefully, others who seem always to be shuffling or stumbling along. There are people who develop resonant and pleasing voices; others whose voices are sharp and grating. There are people who learn to write well; others whose penmanship is far from adequate. It's no less true that many people never learn proper vision habits. Although they may have organically perfect eyes, they see poorly because they use their eyes poorly.

In addition, although they learned to see well originally, many people develop improper habits later, as we'll soon discover.

First, however, it will be most helpful to understand how seeing is achieved.

It's an oversimplification to compare the eye to a camera, as is so frequently done, but the comparison does, at least, offer a reasonable starting point.

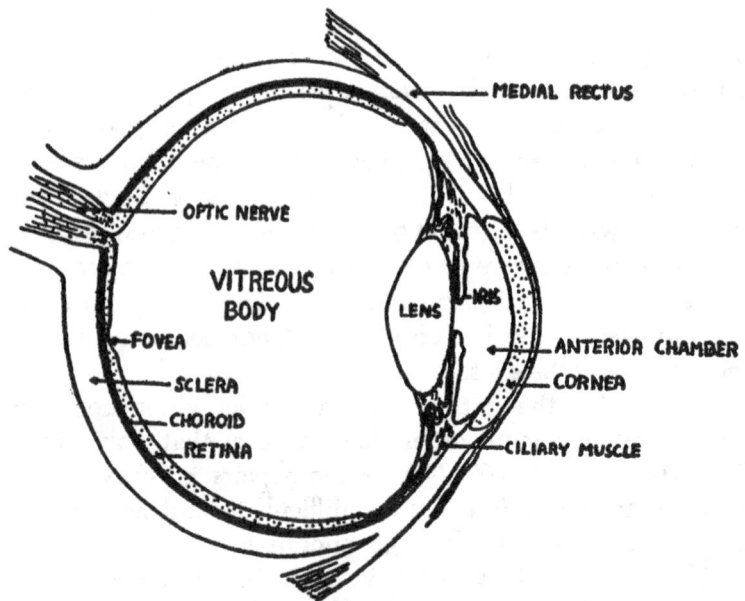

Fig. 2   Diagram of Eye

When you direct a camera at some object, seeking to capture an image of it on film, your objective is to have the light rays, which are always bouncing off the object, enter the camera as you click the shutter open, then pass through a lens which will focus the diffuse rays to a sharp point on the film.

The eye, too, traps and focuses light rays.

In construction, the eye is a three-layered ball. The innermost layer, the retina, is roughly equivalent to film. The middle layer, the choroid, has no equivalent in the camera, since the eye, unlike the mechanical box, needs nourishment, and the choroid is essentially a maze of blood vessels whose function is to feed and enliven the eye. The outermost layer, a tough protective fibrous tissue, known technically as the sclera and popularly as the white of the eye, encompasses the eyeball, opaque everywhere except for a roundish transparent area at the front known as the cornea, or window of the eye. Through here, the light rays enter.

Let's follow them.

Once past the cornea, the rays move through transparent fluid in the front, or anterior, chamber of the eye, arriving next at the iris, a flexible diaphragm with a transparent center, the pupil. As it expands or contracts the pupil, the iris controls the amount of light entering farther into the eye.

Beyond the pupil, the light rays next pass through the lens which refracts or bends them so that, instead of scattering in all directions, they are focused toward the sensitive area of the retina. The focused rays arrive at the retina after one more intermediate journey, through the vitreous body, a transparent, jelly-like substance.

Actually, the retina is not only the innermost layer of the eye but also a continuation of the optic nerve that leads to the brain. If you place your two arms together so that the wrists touch each other, then cup your hands as if you were lightly holding a large bowl, your arms can be likened to the optic nerve and the insides of your hands to the retina lining the eyeball.

The retina contains some forty-five million receptors or nerve endings of two kinds: the rods and cones.

The cones are the more light-sensitive and there is a heavy concentration of them in a small area, yellow in color, known as the macula lutea, slightly off center toward the temples. The very greatest concentration of cones occurs in the fovea centralis, the center of the macula lutea. The rods are concerned with grosser vision and night seeing. The fovea has no rods at all but is made up entirely of cones. Toward the outer portions of the retina there are more rods than cones.

As the rods and cones receive light rays, each minute ending picks up a fraction of the image, converts it into a nerve impulse and transmits it to the brain. The process is something like that used in television.

In the brain, tremendous activity ensues. First, much of the image from the left eye goes to the right lobe of the brain, while much of the image from the right eye goes to the left lobe. Both images then circle around to the back of the brain where they are combined into a single image which continues on to the cortical center. From the cortical center, then, nerve impulses are sent out to regulate accommodation, blinking and other functions which govern the action of the eye in focusing for distance and sharpening the image. Finally, the image goes to the perceptual centers—the reasoning area—where it is analyzed for spatial relations, comparison and contrast, is recognized or remembered—in short, connected up with all of the individual's previous experience, visual and otherwise.

Thus the process of seeing, if all goes well. Far more sensitive and complex than television or any camera—with two eyes working together to produce binocular vision with depth perception!

What can go wrong?

In the most common types of faulty vision, light rays are not sharply focused on the retina and a blur results. When the rays are brought to their sharpest focus in front of, rather than directly on the retina, there is nearsightedness. When the rays are so focused that they come to their sharpest point behind the retina, the result is farsightedness.

What causes defective focusing?

As we've seen earlier, it is the lens of the eye which focuses the light rays. In the nineteenth century, Helmholtz, a great German physiologist, offered the theory that we see distant objects clearly when the lens is flat and relaxed, and we see nearby objects clearly when a muscle, called the ciliary, contracts and in doing so makes the elastic lens bulge out.

But the ability of the ciliary muscle to change the shape of the lens for seeing near objects is limited by the hardness of the lens. A young child can see clearly objects as close as two and a half inches. But with increasing age, as the lens gradually hardens, the limits of close seeing are extended to approximately four inches at age thirty, and to ten inches at age fifty. In later years, as the lens hardens further, most people lose the ability to accommodate their eyes to reading or close working distance. This is presbyopia and it is thus the result of a structural defect in the lens.

Similarly, according to this theory, other structural defects account for other visual deficiences. Just as our bodies vary in length and curvature—people are short or stout or thin or tall—so do our eyes. The farsighted eye is too short; the nearsighted one, too long—too short or too long for even a perfect natural lens to accommodate properly.

In a newborn child, the eye is about 70 per cent of the size it will reach in adulthood. As the child grows, the eye lengthens so that the distance of the retina from the lens increases. If all goes well, if the eye lengthens to the proper extent, it is capable of perfect accommodation. But if the eye lengthens too much, nearsightedness results, or if it doesn't lengthen enough farsightedness must result.

In nearsightedness, farsightedness and presbyopia, the only practical means of improving vision, according to the old theory, is to use glasses to correct for a structural defect in the lens itself or to try to compensate for the structural defect in the shape of the eye by adding to the lens power.

But, at the beginning of the twentieth century, Dr. W. H. Bates, a New York ophthalmologist, began to have doubts that the old theory provided the whole explanation for visual difficulties.

For one thing, he noted in wonderment that in many people, after the lens had been surgically removed, the eye was still capable of accommodation.

In the course of many thousands of eye examinations at the New York Eye and Ear Infirmary and other institutions, he also found that errors of refraction did not remain constant. He learned that even in normal eyes, emotional upsets, poor health, or great strain could cause temporary troubles. From his work, Bates evolved another theory.

When a photographer wants to take a picture of a distant object, he shortens the distance between the lens and the film of the camera. When he wants to take a close-up picture, he lengthens the distance. Bates held that accommodation is accomplished in the same manner in the eye—by a change in shape of the eyeball.

The eyeball is held in its socket by six external muscles. The four recti muscles that reach longitudinally from the socket to the front of the eyeball are concerned with moving the eye to right, to left and up and down. These movements are under your own control. But the same muscles have an involuntary action concerned with pulling back on the eyeball to flatten it when you look at a distant object, thus shortening the distance between lens and retina just as the photographer shortens the distance between lens and film.

There are also two oblique muscles extending around the eyeball. When they squeeze tightly, they lengthen the distance, automatically making the accommodation necessary for seeing at the closest point—for reading a book or for a minute examination of a small object, for example.

A nearsighted person, Bates decided, is one whose oblique muscles are too tight all the time. Consequently, while close point vision is good, distant vision is not because the tightened oblique muscles resist the efforts of the recti muscles to pull the eyeball back, and thus contract or shorten the distance within it sufficiently to accommodate for distance.

The farsighted person is one whose recti muscles are pulling too tightly, resisting the efforts of the oblique muscles to permit accommodation for close point vision.

There are other factors involved, such as the lens. But the action of the muscles is one of the primary requisites for accommodation.

The Bates theory puts a new light on vision difficulties. For if muscle action changes the shape of the eyeball to permit accommodation, it must be remembered that muscle action itself is controlled by nerve impulses. And Bates sought the cause of improper muscle action, or muscle imbalance, in the mind and nervous system.

While poor sight has been held responsible for strain—and, in the end, for fatigue, irritability, nervousness and tension—Bates and his followers came to believe just the reverse: that strain, mental and emotional, can cause poor eyesight.

There is growing awareness today of the integration of mind and body. It's now recognized by the medical profession that many physical disturbances may be brought on or accentuated by emotional problems. In a long list of ailments—including stomach ulcers, heart trouble and high blood pressure—mental and emotional strain is recognized as a frequent prime cause or contributing factor.

The Bates theory, therefore, is not entirely radical when it emphasizes the influence on vision of a factor whose influence elsewhere in the body is well established.

Virtually all adults are subject to continuous tension. Individuals differ in their ability to live with, deal with and relax under strain. One partner in a business firm in financial difficulties may get stomach ulcers while the other partner has no impairment of health. Just so, one person under tension may suffer vision loss while another does not.

In many cases, when children begin school, when they are suddenly thrown into a classroom situation where adjustment to a new way of living is demanded of them, they may develop bad seeing habits as the result of tension and strain. And as they grow older, the tensions of our complex society reinforce bad seeing habits.

In some cases, vision difficulties may have an original physical cause, such as a childhood ailment which temporarily weakens the eyes—as it does the rest of the organism. Emotional tension or shock may contribute to prolong the difficulty and lead to bad seeing habits, which can saddle the child for life as he tries desperately to see what's expected of him.

In a modest little survey, I asked one hundred near-sighted high-school students a series of questions regarding their sight.

1. When did you first notice your loss of sight?
2. What grade were you in then?
3. What subjects did you like?
4. What subjects did you dislike?
5. What kind of lighting did you have in the classroom?
6. Did you take part in sports?
   a. What sports did you like?
   b. What sports did you dislike?
7. Did you like school?
8. Did you like your teacher?

Answers to all questions but the last varied. On that, eighty-eight out of the hundred questioned made some remark such as this: "She was the only teacher I ever had that I disliked!"

Eighty-two per cent of the farsighted people who have worked with me have told me they had some emotional crisis just before they lost their ability to see at the close point. Their crises included: grief caused by a death in the family, difficulty with a child, marital troubles, worry about someone's alcoholism, anxiety about a son in the war, financial troubles and worry over poor health.

The idea that mental and emotional states may *somehow* play a role has found considerable support among many ophthalmologists.

In 1932, one year after Bates's death, in a paper in the *Journal of the American Medical Association* (99:284), Dr. C. W. Rutherford discussed how nervous factors may be associated with some vision disorders and quoted Emerson who had long before observed that patients should be examined as individuals and not as optical mechanisms to be fitted to a test chart and "that lenses should be fitted to a patient's nervous system as well as his eyes."

In "Emotion and Eye-Symptoms," another paper appearing soon afterward in the *British Journal of Psychology*, the point was made that "The mental and emotional state of the patient has not been considered, and the possibility of this state determining the eye symptoms instead of the eye condition causing the general manifestations appears to have eluded both oculist and physician."

Dr. H. Flanders Dunbar, in her book *Emotions and Bodily Changes* (published for the Josiah Macy, Jr., Foundation by Columbia University Press, New York, 1938) noted: "The last decades of psychology and psychiatry have brought about revolutionary changes in point of view of permanent value in research and clinical practice. Ophthalmology thus far has not taken advantage of the progress made by its sister disciplines. It seems almost as if it had remained out of contact with the vital stream of new knowledge, although many of the findings of psychology and psychiatry are of special interest to ophthalmology."

Recently, in an interview, one of the nation's top ophthalmologists remarked, "Although it is easy to rip all Bates's theories to pieces, he did upset all notions that eyesight is a fixed quantity which can be improved only with glasses. Many of his patients thought they saw better—whether instruments said so or not. And in thinking they saw better, they did see better—for at least half of seeing is in the brain."

It is interesting that in more serious problems, too, vision re-education is often of value. People with cataracts, glaucoma and other serious disorders have been helped to a significant extent by sight retraining. And while there are variations in techniques, the basic ones—including the achievement of relaxation and the relief of tension, the increase in mobility of sight and centralization, the improvement of fusion—are used in all cases.

Let's see, now, the first step in improving vision.

Chapter III

Beginning Rehabilitation: Easing the Eyes

Relaxation can do more than rest your eyes. By relieving strain and tension—mental as well as muscular—it will provide the opening wedge for most easily, quickly and comfortably eliminating poor seeing habits and establishing good ones. It is the first essential step on the road to improving your sight.

In virtually every type of visual difficulty, the relaxation procedures described in this chapter have been found to be helpful. They are simple, pleasant, take relatively little time and can be fitted into the busiest schedule. All are done with glasses off—and without any discomfort; indeed, just the reverse.

1. SUNNING

Sunning, or taking light on the closed lids, is one of the most beneficial of all techniques—useful every day and several times a day.

Except when the sun is out, you will use a 75-, 100- or 150-watt light bulb, taking the illumination from it while you sit comfortably in a chair. If you use a 75-watt bulb, place it about two feet from your eyes. For a 100-watt bulb, the distance should be about three feet; for a 150-watt bulb, three and a half feet. My instructors use a 150-watt reflector spotlight during lessons. If you have one of these, or wish

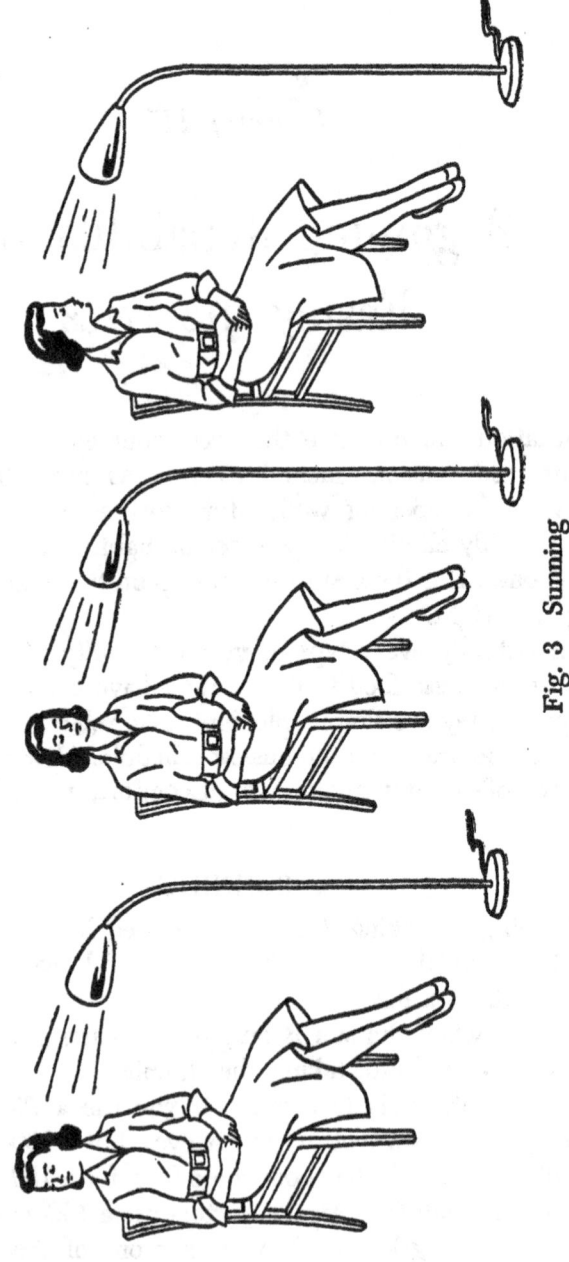

Fig. 3 Sunning

to buy one, start your sunning with the spotlight at eight feet and gradually move it in to six feet from your closed eyes. If you have photophobia and light bothers you, you can sit farther away, in the beginning, from any bulb you use. Gradually, you'll be able to shorten the distance.

Caution: *Never* under any circumstances use a *sun lamp*, heat lamp or fluorescent light on your unprotected eyes.

Sunning should always be done with the eyes *closed*. Open-eyed techniques of sunning have been advocated in the past. But even if not dangerous, brilliant light shining directly into the open eyes is not comfortable—and you can hope for no thorough relaxation, the goal, in the presence of discomfort. Taking the light on your closed lids will be beneficial, and all the more so because you will be comfortable.

With your light in position, seat yourself comfortably in a chair, facing it, eyes closed. Turn your head gently toward your left shoulder. From here, swing it easily toward your right shoulder. Swing back again toward the left and continue to swing back and forth as the illustration shows. You don't tip the head but hold it perfectly poised. Keep the swing short. If you feel even the slightest bit of tension in your neck, you are turning your head too far. The total swing should cover no more than ninety degrees—*toward* but not *to* each shoulder.

As you sun, you should begin to feel a sense of relaxation. You may even feel a little drowsy—and this is good.

You will also get an optical illusion that the light itself is moving—to the right as you swing your head to the left, and vice versa.

Continue sunning with a head motion gently and slowly. Say to yourself lazily as you turn your head, "The light is on my right side. The light is on my left side. The light is on my right side, etc." Say the words slowly to yourself, and you will find that your head motion is slow and easy.

When the sun is out, you can go to a window and take sunlight on your closed eyes with the same head motion. In bright sunlight you will not be able to sun as long as in artificial light. Do it for just a very few minutes at a time. Don't try to overdo.

Practice sunning as often as you can. Try to get a session of it in the morning before you have breakfast and again afterward. Try to do it in the evening before and after dinner, and finally before going to bed.

Have no fears about light. Unfortunately, we are rapidly becoming a nation of sunglass wearers—afraid of light. "The vogue for tinted lenses," an *American Medical Association Journal* report noted, "has reached such an extent that most laymen and many ophthalmologists believe that the eyes need protection not only against daylight but any light, even night light. Informed ophthalmologists disapprove the widespread, continuous and indiscriminate use of tinted lenses and object to the methods and wording of the advertisers of these glasses. A person's toleration of light may be low, and certainly if there is glare from the sands of the desert or the waters of oceans or lakes, or a glare from snow, colored glasses can be worn. But our widespread use of colored glasses must be deplored."

Avoid glare—but don't avoid light.

Sight depends on light. Those of us who cannot live and work out of doors can compensate for our lack of sunshine by taking more light on our closed eyes. Whole squadrons of night bomber pilots during World War II were told to stay out of doors as much as possible during the daytime to renew their acuity of vision for night flying. One former Navy pilot told me that at one time he had difficulty in passing a retest for vision until the doctor in charge told him to step outside, close his eyes and turn his head from side to side in sunlight for two or three minutes. After following the suggestion, he returned to read the eye chart again, this time perfectly.

Sunning is helpful to the mind. Because it is constantly concerned with the shape, color, size, depth and other aspects of objects, the mind can become tired. When the eyes are closed in sunning, there is nothing for the mind to interpret. There is only light. No wonder people find this so mentally restful that they become drowsy.

After the mind has been relaxed to this extent, it is ready to resume its role as the developer or interpreter of what the eyes see and to perform its function with more ease and greater clarity. Nearsighted people often exclaim with surprise at the clearness of a room and its objects—and farsighted people at the clarity of print—when they open their eyes after a few minutes of sunning.

For some time after sunning, you will be aware not only of increased clarity of vision but also of the "good feeling" of your eyes. You will also notice increased relaxation of the whole body. If you're emotionally upset and your neck muscles feel tense, the gentle head motion used in sunning will help to decrease the tension.

Sunning seems to be especially helpful for crossed eyes. One young girl used to seat herself in a comfortable chair for twenty minutes, close her eyes and swing her head from side to side before going to a dance. When I suggested that this might be too much at one time, unless she sat far away from the lamp, she said, "But it feels so good and afterward my eyes stay straight all evening."

2. A VARIATION: PERFORATED
BOARD SUNNING

On a piece of cardboard about 14 inches long by 8 or 9 inches wide, draw horizontal lines an inch apart and vertical lines also one inch apart. At each crossing punch a hole about ⅛ inch in diameter, using an icepick or sharp pencil.

Bring your lamp a little closer to your chair than in regular sunning and hold up the perforated cardboard between you and the lamp, about three inches away from your nose. Close your eyes and swing the board in front of them, using a gentle oval motion (see Fig. 4). After about ten full ovals, bring the cardboard down onto your lap and let the full light shine on your closed lids for a count of ten. Then repeat with the board.

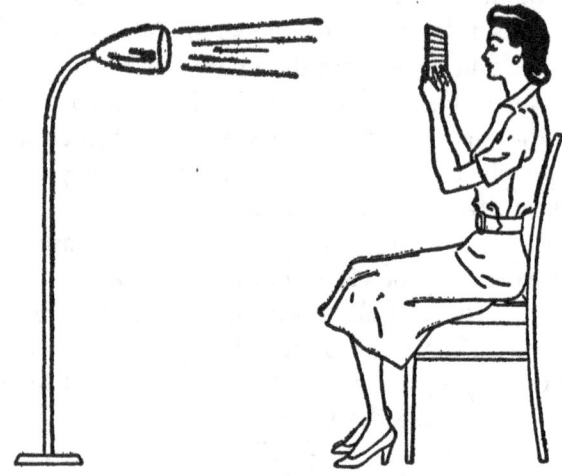

Fig. 4   Perforated Board Sunning

Perforated board sunning produces an effect much like that of sunlight streaming down through the gently moving branches of a tree as you lie beneath it. There is gentle alternation of light and darkness, and it's this which apparently accounts for the effectiveness of the drill.

3. PALMING

The second major aid for relaxation is palming (see Fig. 5). Cup the palms of both hands over your eyes. The fingertips of one hand should be slightly crossed over those of the other on your forehead. Do not stiffen your fingers. Keep them relaxed.

Palm while seated comfortably with both feet on the floor. A pillow on your lap will support your elbows. You should never lean all the way over with elbows on knees; that position makes you tense. If you do not have a large pillow, place your elbows on a table or on a desk in front of you. Your neck should feel relaxed as you lean shoulders and head just slightly forward.

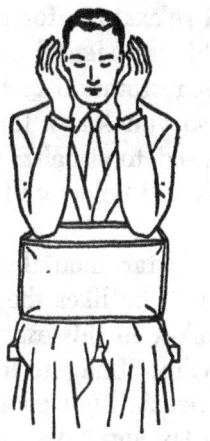 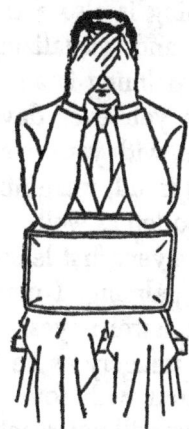

Fig. 5   Palming

Palming while lying down is beneficial, too. One elbow and shoulder should rest against the back of the couch for support.

Close your eyes while palming. Make certain your fingers are loose and do not touch the eyes but that the palms are cupped over them. Never under any circumstances press or rub the eyes. With your eyes closed and the palms over them, no light should come in. And now the complete change from light to darkness should give you a feeling that the eyes are "letting go," losing their tension. Do not try to imagine that you are seeing a uniform field of blackness. While some eye-training schools advise this, it is almost impossible for a beginner to achieve it. You will probably see a black field shot with gray. Later, when your eyes become more relaxed, the field of blackness will come automatically.

Palming helps because of the warmth it brings to the eyes as well as the darkness. Your palms should not be cold when you start. If they feel chilled, let hot water run over them for a brief period. Eyes that are so tense that they have a vision loss may suffer from poor circulation. The warmth of the hands should increase circulation.

Palming is also a time for mental relaxation, for remembering and visualizing pleasant things. Mental imagery during palming is an important sight restoration technique.

Have you ever daydreamed? If so you know that it is possible, with your eyes opened or closed, to visualize objects in your mind, imagining their shapes and colors and seeing their motion as well.

In the very first lesson at my studio, I start mental imagery during palming. I may ask a student if he likes the ocean. If the answer is yes, I ask him to follow in this example of mental imagery as he continues to palm: "Imagine that you are seated with some friends on a beach, high enough up so waves will not reach you. On your lap you have a copy of a magazine. It's a warm, sunny day. Can you feel the warmth of the sun? The sky is very blue. Can you see its blueness?" Usually, he can. If there's difficulty, a repetition usually is successful.

Then I continue: "The water is very blue, too. And now, as you look out at the blue water, you see waves rolling in. One breaks in a pile of white foam and you watch the foam racing up the sand toward you—and then see the tentacles of foam being pulled back into the sea. Can you see all that?

"Now you glance down again and read your magazine. Then you glance up again and watch another wave come in. And here come a little boy and a little girl up near you and your friends. The little boy has a big red and white beach ball. He is toward your left and the girl is to your right. The boy throws the ball, which passes in front of you, and the girl catches and throws it back to him. They continue to toss it back and forth. Can you see the ball going through the air?"

By this time the student looks much more relaxed. He has been able to follow it all, see it all in his mind, more and more readily, and continues to do so as I go on.

"Look out again and see another wave come in slowly at first but with a final rush of power. Notice again how blue the water is. Look out beyond the breaking surf to where some people are swimming. One is wearing an orange-colored swimming cap which stands out in bright contrast against the blue water. Now watch another wave come in. Glance down again to your magazine and mentally read a few words. Now turn to look at the boy. Watch him toss the ball to the girl. Look at the white surf, out to the orange swimming cap, and then extend your sight out to a white sailboat.

"The hull of the boat you see now is black, but the sails are white, and standing in front of the sails there's a man in jeans and red sweater. Now watch a new wave come in, glance down at the magazine, watch the ball go from the boy to the girl, then watch another wave come in, and after it pulls back into the sea, note how dark the sand is where it was moistened. Now look out to the orange-colored swimming cap and off to the sailboat, then even farther out, all the way out to the horizon where you see an ocean liner."

Then I ask him to drop his hands, open his eyes and glance, with a head motion, around the room. In most cases, a look of incredulity appears as the student notes how much brighter color seems and how much more clearly objects in the room stand out.

One of the most successful teachers I ever trained added other senses to her drills in mental imagery. If she took people in their minds to the mountains, she had them mentally dip their hands in a mountain stream and feel its coolness. She had them smell the odor of wood smoke or of coffee.

You can use many pleasant past experiences in practicing mental imagery while palming. Here are just a few examples: a walk in the park; a trip to the mountains; a trip through a department store; a browsing walk through city streets; a hunting or camping trip; a visit to a circus. You can do a mental "run-through" of a movie or TV program.

In your practice, visualize in color and motion, see things at all distances, near and far. If you're nearsighted, pay particular attention to distant imagery; if you're farsighted, emphasize visualization at the close point. If you're cross-eyed, try to visualize with depth perception.

The person with normal sight has no difficulty in mental visualization. He can see clearly, in his mind, an object in the distance and then one close to him. He has good mental as well as physical accommodation. Many, if not most, people with poor sight have difficulty in mental visualization at first. Rebuilding your ability for mental imagery is a valuable aid in restoring sight.

Do not be alarmed if you cannot visualize perfectly in the beginning. Your ability to visualize may have been lost slowly over a period of many years. It will return, with practice and the help of relaxation techniques, much more quickly.

Palming and mental imagery practice are more beneficial if done in numerous short periods rather than in one long period. Set aside a few minutes at various times of the day for practice. Stick to this schedule. Make palming and imagery a part of your daily life.

4. ALTERNATE SUNNING AND PALMING

Both sunning and palming, excellent techniques for achieving relaxation when used alone, are even more effective when used in combination. Then, each seems to enhance the effect of the other. Whenever possible, follow a period of sunning with a period of palming.

There are benefits to be derived, too, from practice in alternate sunning and palming. Sit in front of your light at the regular distance and place on your lap the pillow you use for palming or, if you use desk or table for palming, sit in front of that. Take the light on your closed lids for the count of ten, then palm for a count of ten. Sun again, then palm again, and continue doing so alternately for a few minutes.

The quick succession of light and darkness will prove restful and relaxing. It's helpful, too, in overcoming any difficulty you may have in seeing clearly when you move from light to darkness or vice versa.

5. THE LONG SWING

First used by Dr. Bates, the long swing is an excellent method of increasing relaxation of the whole body. As illustrated in Fig. 6, you stand straight and at ease, without stiffness, with your feet parallel to each other. They should be about twelve inches apart if you are five feet, five inches tall. If you're shorter, bring your feet a little closer together; if taller, place them farther apart. Experiment until you have found the stance that is most comfortable for you.

With your arms hanging loosely at your sides and your head level, swing your whole body in a turn to the left and then to the right, shifting your weight from one foot to the other as you do so. As you swing to the left, your right heel should come up slightly; as you swing right, your left heel should be raised. The whole swing should make an arc of 180 degrees. You can check on this by noting, before you start, the side walls of the room at points opposite your shoulders. Do not turn beyond these points.

Stand facing a window, if possible. As you swing from side to side, let your gaze drift along with the swing, from one side of the room, across and out the window, then on to the

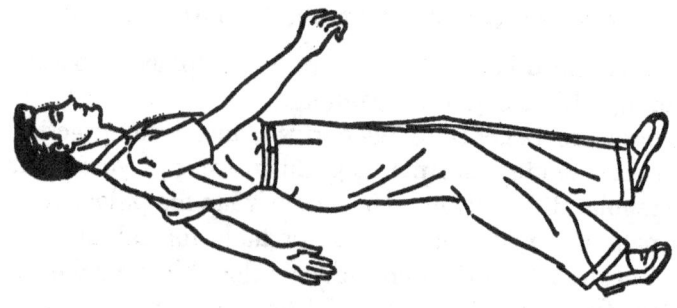

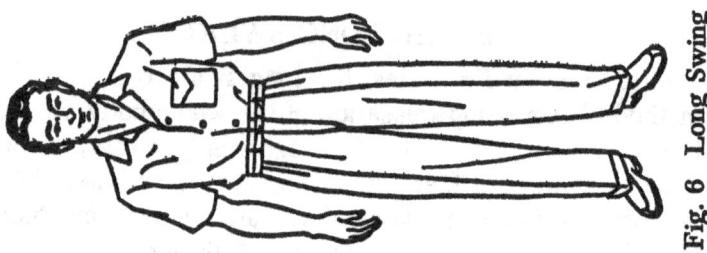

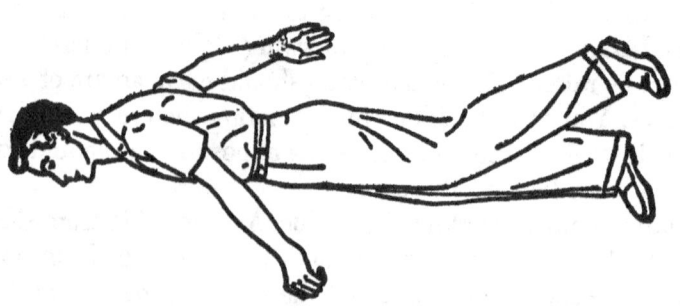

Fig. 6 Long Swing

other side of the room. Except for blinking, the gaze should follow an imaginary horizontal eye-level line continuously—with no jumps from one object to another, no gaps in your seeing.

You should soon get the optical illusion that the window-frames are moving in a direction opposite to your swing while objects outside the window—buildings or trees, for example—are moving in unison with you. It's an interesting illusion, and when you achieve it you know you're doing the long swing properly.

Use your record player or radio for rhythm and to help keep the swing slow. A Strauss waltz will give you perfect timing.

If the swing makes you dizzy, you are staring, not letting your gaze move along freely and easily. Stop for a moment and try again.

One caution: If your doctor has ordered you to avoid physical activity, do not do the long swing without his permission.

Remember that the swing is for basic bodily relaxation. The movement is easy, gentle and slow. If you do it fast and vigorously, you are doing an "exercise" that will not benefit your sight.

Done properly, the long swing will bring a restful sensation to the eyes and make your whole body feel more relaxed. It's also valuable because it helps to break any staring habit which, as we will see in Chapter IV, is a frequent factor in many types of vision loss.

Many of my students have found the long swing excellent just before going to bed at night. Because of the general bodily relaxation it induces, it seems to help many people troubled with insomnia. Some students have used it when they've waked up during the night and been unable to go back to sleep. Four or five dozen long swings, they report, have helped them fall asleep again without further difficulty.

Another important benefit comes from long-swing practice just before retiring for the night. Have you ever had the experience of waking up in the morning, after what had seemed to be a good night's sleep, only to find your eyes feeling tired? The cause may have been that your eyes were not in a relaxed state when you went to sleep and stayed tense, staring under the lids all during the night. The long swing helps avoid such tension and staring.

6. SHORT SWINGS

The following short swings, all done with the eyes closed, are excellent aids to relaxation. They help ease tension in neck muscles and, in the process, may bring about better circulation which aids vision. Many can be done inconspicuously and there will be frequent opportunities during the day, at work and play, when you can practice one or more of them without attracting undue attention.

THE SUNNING SWING

This is the same swing you use in sunning. With eyes closed, move your head horizontally in a short arc—two to three inches to the left, then front, and two to three inches to the right, and then to front again. Avoid speed and jerks of the head. All of the benefit comes from the slow, gentle motion.

THE VERTICAL SWING

Begin with your head facing straight ahead. Then, slowly and gently, with eyes closed, lift your head up two to four inches and bring it down until your chin almost rests on your chest. Continue up and down, making certain that you are not holding your head stiffly and that the motion is gentle, slow and continuous. You should feel—in this swing and all the others—that your neck muscles are relaxing, "letting go."

THE CIRCULAR SWING

Lift your head up two inches, and from this starting point describe a small clockwise circle, imagining that you are using your nose to draw a line in the air, the circumference of the circle. Remember to make it a small circle and to keep the motion slow, gentle, continuous.

After forming six or eight circles with a clockwise motion, reverse and make another six or eight counter-clockwise.

THE X-SWING

Move your head slowly and gently a short distance up and to the right. Imagine, as you do this, that you are using your nose to draw a line from the center of a clock face to the two o'clock position. From the two o'clock position, move your head down toward the center again and then on to the eight o'clock position. Go back from here to center. Repeat this motion three times.

Next, starting again from the imaginary center of the clock, move your head to the ten o'clock position. From there, proceed to the four o'clock position, then back to center. Do this three times.

Begin the first part again and repeat the entire drill six or eight times. In combination, the lines you've formed make an X.

THE LAZY-DAISY SWING

Move your head gently and slowly so that, using your nose like an imaginary pencil, you form a complete circle toward your left. Then, form a second circle to your right. The two circles combined make a figure 8 lying on its side.

Now, move your head upward to form a small circle. Then move it downward to form another small circle. This combination will give you a figure 8 standing up.

As you repeat this drill, first moving to left and right, then up and down, forming the two figures 8, you will get the sensation that you are making a four-leaf daisy.

It is best to do each figure 8 several times before trying to combine the two.

THE COGWHEEL SWING

Picture in your mind an ordinary cogwheel—a circular wheel with scalloped edges—such as you will find inside your watch.

In this drill, you move your head in a circular motion to form a complete wheel, outlining as you go the scallops on the wheel. From the starting position, with head pointing straight ahead, move straight up and, beginning here, at the top of the imaginary wheel, move clockwise, form a scallop, move clockwise some more and form another scallop, until you've gone around to make the whole wheel. Do this three or four times, then reverse and go counter-clockwise.

It's the extra little motion involved in forming the scallops that makes this swing of great benefit.

All the short swings are valuable but all need not be done each day. You will find that your step-by-step program will call for one or two daily. Vary them. In the program, too, you will find a guide for when to use the other relaxation techniques given in this chapter.

Chapter IV

Acquiring Centralized
Vision and Mobility

If you wished to feel the texture of an object, you would use your fingertips rather than your knuckles or palms—the most sensitive areas of your hands rather than areas capable only of gross feeling. And for clearest vision, it is just as essential to use a part of the eye which is designed for fine rather than gross sensitivity. Learning to do this—at all times —will take you a long step forward in improving your sight —no matter what your problem is.

You'll remember from Chapter II that the retina of the eye is sensitive to light, but there is one area in its center, the fovea centralis, which is most sensitive. Only the part of an image falling upon the fovea can be seen most clearly while other parts, picked up elsewhere on the retina, will be somewhat blurred.

The fovea is so tiny that, with perfect sight, you can see clearly, at one time, at reading distance, an area only about the size of a dime. At a distance of twenty feet, the area will be only about two and a half inches in diameter.

Nature, it would seem, meant vision to be a pinpointing process involving great mobility, with the eyes constantly shifting to take in large images in small, clear segments. Movement, indeed, is essential in the use of all the senses. As the French psychologist T. A. Ribot has noted: "If we keep . . . our eyes fixed on any one single point, after a while our vision becomes confused; a cloud is formed between the object and ourselves, and finally we see nothing at all. If we lay our hand flat upon a table motionless and without pressure (for pressure itself is a movement), by slow degrees the sensation wears off and finally disappears. The reason is that there is no perception without movement, be it ever so weak."*

People lose sight when they stare fixedly, trying to force vision, to see too much at once. Mobility and central fixation should be normal, unconscious habits. But in some cases, they may not be learned properly during infancy and childhood. In others, they may be lost.

In the last few years, you may have noticed that the print in books for children has become larger and larger—in some, printed letters are half an inch or an inch high. If the area that can be seen by the fovea centralis at reading distance is only about dime size, how can a child's eyes see clearly a whole word, even a word of only three letters, when each letter is as tall as the diameter of a dime? This large print, which could possibly cause loss of centralization, may be at least a partial reason for poor sight in some children.

Loss of mobility and centralized vision may come, too, when sight begins to deteriorate from other causes. For example, if there is some loss of accommodation or fusion, the individual may make great but mistaken efforts to buck up his sight by peering hard, staring fixedly, trying mightily to force better vision. As he does this, mobility is lost, centralized vision is not used and, in a vicious cycle, vision is further impaired.

However lost, mobility and centralized sight can be regained by the simple techniques that follow. They are aimed, first, at improving mobility. Happily, as mobility increases, as you learn to shift the gaze quickly, you will be

---

* Ribot, T. A., *The Psychology of Attention* (New York: Marcel Rodd Co., 1946), p. 11.

achieving centralization at the same time. Following this, it will be easier to "fine" the centralization, and techniques for achieving this will be given.

You will be rewarded as you do this work by flashes of beautifully clear sight—short episodes in which your potential vision will be experienced. They're gratifying interludes which will boost your morale and encourage you to continue to the point where the flashes are replaced by continuous good vision.

As you practice these techniques, too, you may note a desirable extra dividend. Every time the eyes move, a slightly different picture is recorded in the brain which is able, when called upon to do so, to interpret these pictures with wonderful facility and speed. As you speed sight, there seems to be a speed-up of mental functioning. Many of my students, after a few weeks of practice, have reported that they feel mentally more alert and, even more specifically, they note better comprehension and more retentive memory.

1. COUNTING

As you develop curiosity, you develop motion. Counting is an excellent aid.

Recently a nearsighted woman brought her normally sighted husband to watch one of her lessons. It was his first time in my office and her fourth time. When I asked them both to close their eyes and tell me how many pictures there were in the room, she confessed she didn't know but he gave the correct answer without hesitation. He had the curiosity which is an attribute of normal sight. Increase curiosity and you will improve your sight. For curiosity will help develop mobility.

Start counting right now. Look up, with head as well as eye motion, and count the number of pictures in your room. Look around the room and find all the bits of any shade of red that you can see. Perhaps one of the pictures has some red in it. Maybe there are shades of red in the carpet. Have you checked the drapes? How about books? Do any of them have red bindings? Is there red on the cover of a magazine?

Now take another color—and a third and fourth. You will be surprised at the amount of reds and blues and greens and yellows around you.

You can count colors on advertisements in subway cars and buses. As you practice this color counting drill, you may find within a few days, if you are nearsighted, that you can begin to read some of the letters in the signs. One of my students, a secretary with 20/500 vision, would take off her glasses during her hour's ride in the subway even though she "wouldn't see anything." As she practiced counting colors, she began to see a few isolated letters in signs. Now, a year later, according to her doctor, her vision tests 20/40.

Normal sight is very mobile, and every bit of practice you get in increasing mobility will be important in speeding sight improvement.

Here are more examples of things you can count:

1. Books between bookends
2. Books in a bookcase
3. Objects on a table or desk
4. Top lights on taxicabs at night
5. Hats in a milliner's window
6. Red ties in a haberdasher's window
7. Letters in a sign
8. Windows in a building
9. Trees in a park
10. Branches on a tree
11. Children in a playground
12. People in a room
13. Flowers of one color in a garden
14. Ships in a harbor
15. Pigeons on a sidewalk

2. EDGING

"Edging," another effective method of gaining mobility, simply means looking around the edges of an object, outlining it with a head motion. Look up from this book now and move your head as you look all around the frame of a picture. Look around the four outer sides of the mat and then around the four inner sides. Edge a table in the distance. As you practice edging, you will find that objects become cleaner cut. The hazy lines around them seem to decrease. You are moving your eyes, eliminating staring and, as you move them with head motion, you are pointing them so you use centralized vision, bringing the fovea into use.

Practice edging out of doors. Look up and down the sides of buildings, around the frames of some of the windows. If you are riding, look around the sides of houses and barns in the distance.

Here is just a partial list of an endless number of objects you can edge:

1. Letters on a big sign
2. Candlesticks
3. Furniture
4. Flowers in a bouquet
5. Sides of a country lane
6. Patterns in an Oriental rug
7. Chocolates in a box
8. Articles in a store window
9. Stars and stripes in a flag
10. A human face
11. Shoulders and heads of persons seated ahead of you in a bus or train

After some practice, you will begin to edge without conscious effort and sight will improve.

3. TREE LIGHTS

Do you have a string of Christmas tree lights? You can use them as an extra aid to create habits of mobility. Tie a string of five bulbs to a yardstick, prop the ends of the stick on four or five books set up at each end of a desk or table (see Fig. 7). Plug in and light the bulbs and, in rhythm to

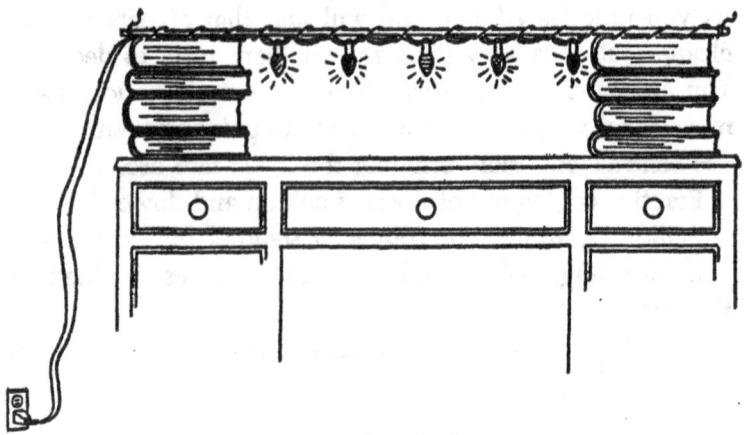

Fig. 7 Tree Lights

music, look from one light to another, turning your head as you do so. At first, you may have only an over-all glimpse of a red bulb, then a green, blue and yellow one. As you continue, you'll find you can outline each light bulb quickly before turning to the next one. Use a right, left, right, left head motion. Look at bulbs one and two, one and two, one and two, next, close your eyes and remember the colors of one and two and continue the head motion, while your eyes are closed. Then open and look and they will now seem to be a little clearer. Go on to look, with the same rhythm, at one and three, two and three, two and three, close and remember, then open and look again at two and three. Continue on in the same fashion with the other bulbs.

4. LIGHTS AND MIRROR

You can achieve mobility at increased distance by setting your tree lights on a table placed in front of a mirror. Put the table as far away from the mirror as you can see the reflected lights without strain or effort. Look from light one to light two in front of you, with a lateral head motion. Then look in the same way at the reflection of lights one and two in the mirror. Look back at lights two and three in front of you, moving from one to the other, and then at the reflections of these lights in the mirror. After some practice, you'll be able to outline the reflected lights quickly as you turn from one to another.

If the lights in the mirror seem vastly enlarged or if a single light seems to be broken up into segments of light and dark, close your eyes for a moment, remember how the lights looked directly in front of you, then open and you'll find that the reflected lights appear clearer.

As you continue to do this drill, you will be able to increase the distance.

5. TOSSING A BALL

Toss a ball from hand to hand. Your head should move naturally as your eyes follow the ball. Now toss it up in the air and watch it as it comes down. This time your head should go up and down as your eyes follow the ball.

When you have become proficient in tossing, throw the ball against a wall in the distance. Let it bounce on the floor before you catch it. Follow it with your eyes. You are speeding your sight. If you can find someone with a sight loss to work with you in exchange for your help to him, play catch or Ping-pong together as often as you can.

Watching ball games is also very good for you. Whenever you go to one, keep your eyes on the ball, following it with a head motion. Take the time to stop and watch for a few minutes whenever you see children playing ball.

6. BLINKING

Blinking is an aid to mobility. It helps to prevent staring. There's no need to blink constantly. A rate of five to seven times a minute is desirable. If you count to ten and then blink, count to ten and blink again, you will see how frequently your lids should close. Close them lightly, easily. Do not pop the eyes open and shut. Practice this until it becomes an unconscious habit.

7. RING SHIFT

Make a ring, like that shown in Fig. 8, by shaping a black wire coat hanger into a circle. On the wire, wrap small pieces of white adhesive tape one inch apart.

Hold the ring about fourteen to fifteen inches in front of your eyes and, *with a circular head motion,* flick your gaze over the black and white intersections. Go around twice, clockwise. Then close your eyes and continue the swing, remembering the intersections as they looked with your eyes open. Open your eyes and go around twice again. Now reverse your head swing and go around the intersections of the ring, counter-clockwise, twice with eyes open, twice with them closed and twice with them open again. The head should be in motion even when the eyes are closed.

8. RULER SHIFT

If you're farsighted, hold a twelve-inch ruler out in front of you at a distance of twelve to fifteen inches. If you're nearsighted, hold it farther away, even at arm's length. In either case, the ruler should be about two inches below the level of your eyes. Its marked edge should be up, and the number 6 on it should be directly in front of your nose (see Fig. 9).

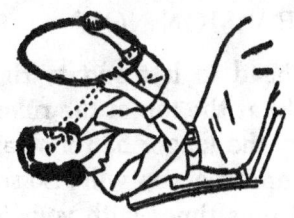

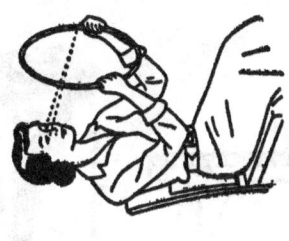

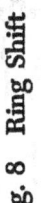

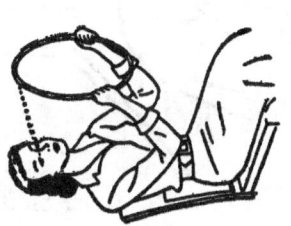

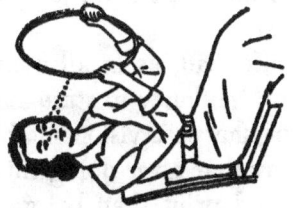

Fig. 8   Ring Shift

Move your head to left and to right, sliding your gaze across the marks at the top of the ruler. At first, you may be able to see only the longer half-inch and inch marks. Later, as your sight improves, you will also see the finer marks.

Do this drill four times with your eyes open. Then do it four times, with speed and rhythm, with eyes closed, remembering the marks. Now, open your eyes again, and as you do the drill four times more, you will notice that the marks seem clearer.

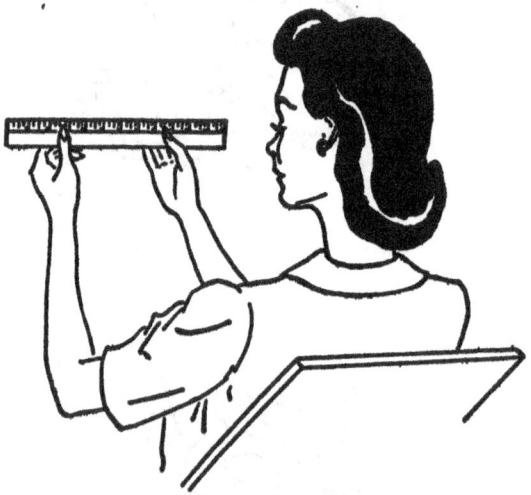

Fig. 9   Ruler Shift

A good variation is to hold the ruler vertically instead of horizontally in front of you, with the top of the ruler sufficiently above eye level so that the 6 will be just in front of your nose. This time, use a vertical head motion to go up and down the ruler.

In this ruler shift drill, as in all mobility drills, you will be overcoming any tendency to stare and making increasing use of the area of sharpest vision in the retina. Farsighted people often report that after doing this drill they can read slightly smaller-sized print than before.

A third variation is to hold the ruler out diagonally in front of you, as if you were using it to connect the figures 2 and 8 on a clock face. Once again, run your eyes with a head motion up and down the ruler four times, close your eyes and repeat, then open and repeat again. Do the drill again with the ruler held as if you were connecting the figures 10 and 4 on a clock face.

9. YARDSTICK SHIFT

Using a yardstick to do the same shifting described in the previous technique is especially helpful for people with glaucoma and retinitis pigmentosa and others who have lost some peripheral vision so they tend to see only small areas in front and little on the sides.

The extra length encourages further "reaching out" to the periphery and hence helps widen the area of sight.

10. SMALL RED SHIFTER

Across a 3 × 5 unruled white file card, ⅛ of an inch from the top, draw a horizontal red line. Then draw vertical red lines ⅛ of an inch apart, extending from the horizontal red line to the top edge of the card.

If you are farsighted, hold the card out one foot in front of you and just a little below eye level. If you're nearsighted, hold the card out at arm's length.

Start at the left edge and run your gaze, with a head motion, to the right across the vertical red lines. Note the lines in passing but do not stop to stare at each one. Make your shift slow but continuous, without pauses. When you reach the right edge of the card, go back again, with a head motion, toward the left edge.

Go from left to right and right to left four times.

Now repeat the drill four times with eyes closed, picturing the red lines in your mind.

Finally open your eyes, repeat again, and you will note that the lines have become a little clearer.

11. LARGE RED SHIFTER

On a piece of white cardboard or heavy white paper, two feet long and five inches wide, draw vertical pencil lines from the top to bottom edge at half-inch intervals. With a red crayon, color in the area between the left edge of the card and the first penciled line. Leave the next half-inch area blank, and color in the third. Continue this across the card so that you have alternate red and white stripes. If you prefer, you can paste on strips of red paper instead of coloring in the stripes.

Use the large red shifter just as you did the small, placing it as far away as you can see it. You may have to start with it propped up just a few feet away. If your sight is extremely poor, you may have to hold it out only a few inches from your eyes. But as you practice with it, and as you use other techniques for improving your vision, you will be able to move it farther and farther out.

12. VERTICAL SHIFT

In many people with vision problems, there is a tendency for the eyes to pull toward the temples. The pull may be slight, hardly noticeable. Exophoria, as the condition is known, is discussed more fully in the next chapter on fusion for it is part of the fusion problem. Vertical shifting, even as it increases mobility, also helps overcome the exophoria tendency, contributing to better fusion, one of the essentials for good sight. It thus has a double value.

There are many ways in which you can practice vertical shifting. You can gaze out the window of your room and, with a vertical head motion, look up and down the edge of the building across the street. You can look up and down the drape at the window. You can run your gaze, too, always with a head motion, up and down the edge of a door, or the edge of a pencil or ruler held in front of your nose.

You'll find many other ways by which, at odd moments during the day, you can get in some valuable practice in vertical shifting.

13. TOSSING DICE

Toss out a pair of dice on a desk or table and, with a head motion, let your gaze follow them as they bounce and turn until they finally come to rest. Try, with brief flashing looks, to see the markings as the dice roll. If you fail now, never mind. The value of this drill lies in the motion.

Roll out the dice and follow them and gather them up and roll them out again. A few minutes of this will be most helpful in making your sight more mobile.

Practice a long roll, too. You might want to do this on the floor. When the dice become more widely separated as they roll out, you'll get a greater range of motion as you shift your gaze from one to the other in following them.

Start with just a pair of dice. As you become more proficient, you can use three, four and five dice, rolling them out all at once but shifting your gaze quickly from one to the other as you follow them.

14. TOSSING CARDS

This is an excellent aid for mobility at desk distance. Shuffle a pack of playing cards, hold it in the palm of one hand and toss a card out to the right of a desk or table. As it falls face up, call it. Toss the next to the left side, and call it as it falls. Continue, tossing in every direction.

You can use this same drill for mobility at greater distance. Stand next to the desk or table and throw and call ten cards. Then move back a foot and throw and call another ten. Move back another foot and throw and call another ten.

15. PLAYING SOLITAIRE

Playing solitaire is good practice for mobility and centralization. Play your game as you ordinarily would. Make sure you turn your head as you look from one card to another. Don't stare. Keep your gaze moving. Occasionally glance up and look off into the distance.

16. "FINING"

All the techniques already given for mobility help at the same time to improve centralization, or the use of the area for "clearest" vision in the retina. As your sight improves, you can practice "fining" your centralization by working with smaller and smaller objects, parts of objects and individual letters in a printed word.

I have had nearsighted people, for example, who at first could only outline the huge form of a tree. After practice, they could outline individual *leaves* of the same tree.

Here are more suggestions for fining:

1. From the over-all design in a cloth to its texture, the arrangement of its threads
2. From a stairway to the individual treads
3. From a number of hats in a milliner's window to the individual flowers on the hats
4. From the books in a case to the designs on the individual book jackets
5. From the large designs in an Oriental rug to the smaller ones
6. From a chair to the fine bits of carving on it
7. From the columns on a public building to the Doric or Corinthian design at the top of each column
8. From the house in the distance to the "gingerbread" decorations on the house
9. From the door to the doorknob

10. From the ashtray to the monogram in the ashtray
11. From the paneling in the wall to the design in the paneling
12. From a person's face to the twinkle in his eye

17. PATCHING

The use of an eye patch, obtainable at any drugstore, is helpful in making certain that you build up the sight of a weaker eye. When you play solitaire, for example, patch the strong eye and play a full game with the weak eye. Then, take off the patch, look around for a moment before patching the other eye and play half a game with the stronger eye. Then remove the patch and finish the second game with both eyes together.

Use a patch some of the time when you count, edge, work with the tree lights and when you toss dice and cards. Use it in "fining," too. Again, as in solitaire, favor the weaker eye by patching the strong one for half the drill, remove the patch and look around for a moment, patch the other eye for the next one-fourth of the drill, then finish with both eyes. Look straight ahead or slightly toward the nose when you use a patch.

Chapter V

Improving Fusion
for Better Vision

Since your eyes are two or more inches apart, measuring from pupil to pupil, each eye sees any object from a slightly different angle. In the brain, the two images are fused, or merged into a single clear image.

If all goes well!

But imperfect fusion is common in all types of vision loss. When it is not a factor in the original loss itself, it may contribute to further deterioration. It may produce discomfort as well.

The improvement of fusion is one of the most important aids to re-establishing good sight—not only to a greater extent than might otherwise be possible but with greater speed and comfort as well.

While the actual process of fusion is mental, it becomes possible only when the eyes transmit to the brain two images that lend themselves to fusion.

Have you ever looked through a stereopticon, an instrument designed to produce the appearance of solidity and relief by combining the images of two similar pictures of an object? Not just any two pictures will do. The combination, or merging, becomes possible only with two carefully chosen pictures. That is equally true in the brain.

To transmit fusible images, the eyes must be properly

directed toward the object you wish to see. If the object is less than twenty feet away, the eyes must converge upon it, turning slightly inward, each at the same angle. Beyond twenty feet, they must look out in parallel. Any deviation may interfere with fusion.

When the deviation is extreme, as in some cross-eyed people, with the eyes far out of alignment, the image from one eye may be suppressed by the mind, except for some side vision. If the deviation is great and one of the images is not suppressed, the result is double vision—two objects seen in place of one.

But lesser deviations, produced by slight imbalance in the muscles which control the movements of the eye, are far more common. Then, the image in the brain may appear only slightly blurred—the edges of a letter, for example, may be fuzzy or the print at the close point may be gray or even slightly double. People with fusion loss sometimes report that the eyes feel strained—hot, tired, gritty, reddened and watery—and a dull ache may occur. The strain may result from both the abnormal muscular pull and the mind's earnest attempts to interpret blurred images.

Something else may happen, too.

When muscular imbalance interferes with proper pointing of the eye, the light rays may go off normal course as they enter and impinge, not on the sensitive central area of the retina, but on the less sensitive portions. If this continues long enough, the center-seeing part of the eye may become dull from lack of use.

Perhaps everyone's fusion goes off balance for brief periods. Excessive drinking, for example, may produce loss of fusion with blurring and double images. Unusual physical stress or nervous tension can also disrupt muscular coordination in the eyes.

In our modern civilization, we seem to have developed a great deal of exophoria. Notice that many of the people you meet have more white toward the nasal than toward the temporal side of the eye, so that the eyes tend to diverge rather than converge. Perhaps one explanation is that so much of our seeing is on a horizontal plane. Our ancestors looked up and down almost as much as they looked from side to side. The farmer looked up and down to see if the furrow he was plowing was straight. The seafaring man looked up and down the masts and checked the rigging. People looked to the skies to note changes in weather.

Today, we look up much less. Most of us are busy much of the day indoors, where our looking is largely from side to side—often with a short cut.

If you want to look at any object toward your left, you can—and should—move your whole head to the left in order to see it with both eyes. Nevertheless, without bothering to turn the head, you can glimpse the object out of the corner of your left eye. In our daily work, usually done at high speed, we take many short cuts and a common visual one is the sideward glance which may tend to pull the eye out, producing divergence rather than convergence.

It has taken a long time to realize the importance of *slight* loss of fusion in causing or contributing to vision difficulties. One thing which may have thrown many investigators off the track is the seeming paradox of the near-sighted person who can read fine print. How is this possible unless fusion is perfect? The answer, it was finally realized, is that a single eye may be used for the reading.

To check this, nearsighted people can hold a pencil up before the nose when reading. In looking beyond the pencil at the reading matter, there should be an optical illusion of two pencils. But many see only one pencil, indicating that only one eye is being used.

It is not always possible to tell whether the eyes are working together properly for fusion by observing them in a mirror or having someone else observe them.

But there is a check which will show whether you have good fusion. On a file card, draw two dime-size circles parallel to each other, with their centers about one and a half inches apart. Through the left circle, draw a vertical diameter; through the right, a horizontal diameter. Halfway between the two circles, draw a vertical line extending from top to bottom of the card. Thus:

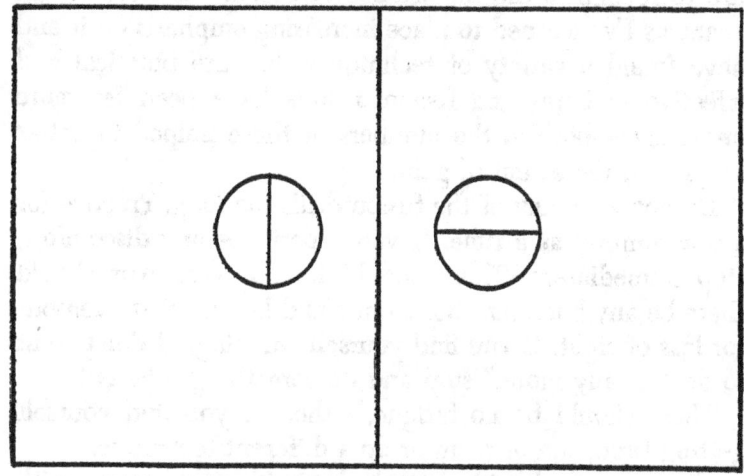

Fig. 10   Fusion Card Check

If you are nearsighted, prop the card three feet away from you. Raise a yardstick with the narrow edge up and place one end of it between your eyes and the other end on the vertical line of the card. Look at the card until you get the optical illusion of two yardsticks extending out from you with a passage between them. Centered in the passage, you should see one circle, with a cross in the center. The horizontal and vertical diameters have merged.

If you're farsighted, use a ruler instead of a yardstick, holding the card at the end of the ruler and proceed in the same way.

If you fail to merge or fuse the circles, the techniques

given below will help to improve your fusion and your vision.

They have proved effective in all types of vision difficulty, including strabismus, or cross-eye.

I have rarely seen a person with a vision difficulty who did not gain great benefit from improving fusion. It is my firm conviction that early instruction in retraining sight—including my own in the first few years—suffered from failure to recognize the importance of fusion. In more recent years, as I've learned to place increasing emphasis on it and have found a variety of techniques that are practical and effective in improving fusion, results have been far more impressive—both in the numbers of those helped to better vision and the extent of gain.

Do not work any of the fusion drills too long. Practice for a few minutes at a time. If you experience any discomfort, stop immediately. There should be no pain. Nor should there be any boredom. Boredom could be one of the reasons for loss of sight. If you find yourself thinking, "I don't want to do this any more," stop and do something different.

There should be no fatigue, either. If you find yourself getting tired, sun or palm or do a different technique.

If you can work with rhythm, do so. Playing a record with a heavy beat is helpful.

It's a good idea, too, to start working these drills in front of a mirror so you can see whether you are doing them properly, which means directly in front of your nose.

1. CORD FUSION

You will need only a twenty-foot length of cord for this. Tie one end to a doorknob or to a chair at some distance from the front of the chair where you'll seat yourself. The tied end should be slightly lower than the level of your eyes in your seated position. Sit down in the chair, directly facing the tied end of the cord. Hold your end of the cord one foot from your eyes. (See Fig. 11.)

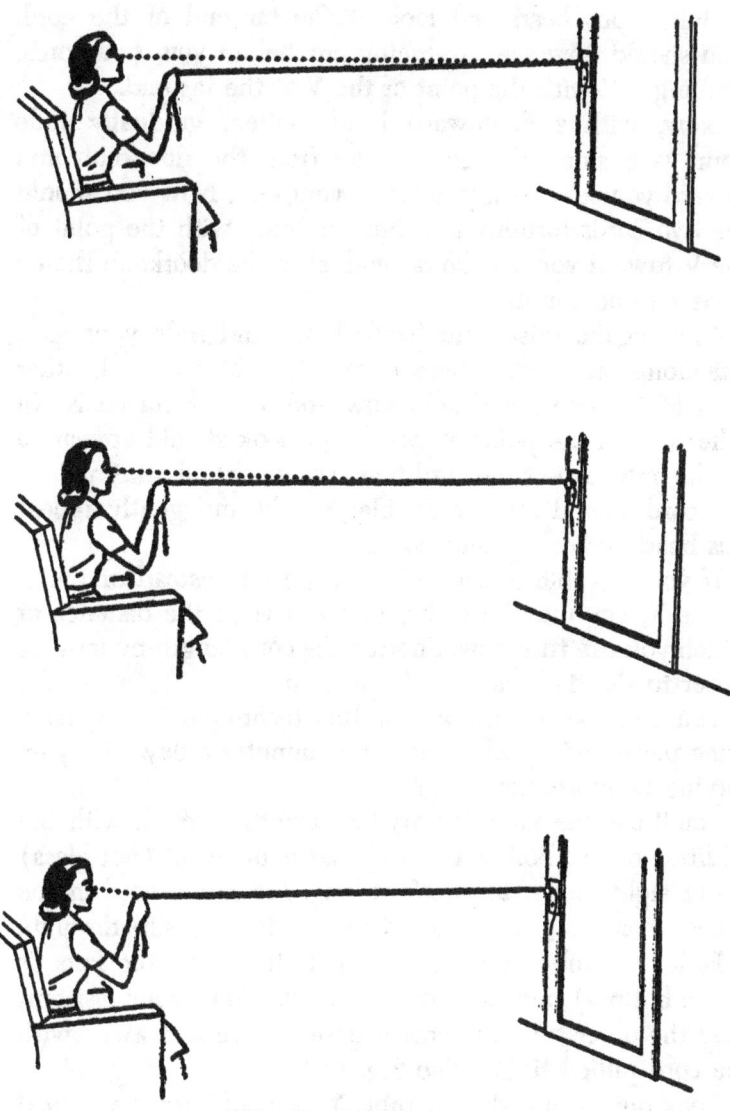

Fig. 11 Cord Fusion

Raise your head and look at the far end of the cord. You should now see, stretching out before you, two cords, forming a V with the point of the V at the far end.

Now, with a downward head motion, gradually slide your gaze along the cord, away from the doorknob and toward yourself, until you reach your end. Now you should see two cords forming a V but this time with the point of the V toward you. At the far end, even the doorknob should appear to be double.

Once again, raise your head slowly and slide your gaze out along the cord. Wherever you look at the cord, other than at the ends, it should now appear to form an X. In other words, the point at which you look should appear to be the only area of the cord that is single; at all other points, the cord should appear double. Slowly and gently repeat this head motion up and down.

If you are able to see only a reverse Y instead of the V or the X, you may be trying to see beyond the distance at which you can fuse now. Shorten the cord length by moving closer to the tied end and begin again.

You can use a variation of this technique if you have some person who will spend a few minutes a day with you, serving as an assistant.

You'll use the same twenty-foot length of cord, with the addition of two hollow tubes of plastic or metal (not glass) about eight inches to one foot long. Insert the cord in the tubes, then knot each end so the cord won't slip through.

Hold one tube vertically, with its top end (the knot is at the bottom) between your eyebrows. Have your assistant hold the other tube in vertical position five feet away with the cord pulled tight. (See Fig. 12.)

Look out toward the far tube. You should get the optical illusion that two cords are extending from your eyes, making a V with the point at the top of the distant tube. Your assistant should hold his end of the cord slightly below your eye level. (Never direct the eyes upward without moving the head up. The natural focus of the eye is slightly down.) The cord should also be held out directly in front of your nose. If your assistant pulls it to one side, you must move your head and point your nose in that direction so that your eyes are looking straight ahead at all times.

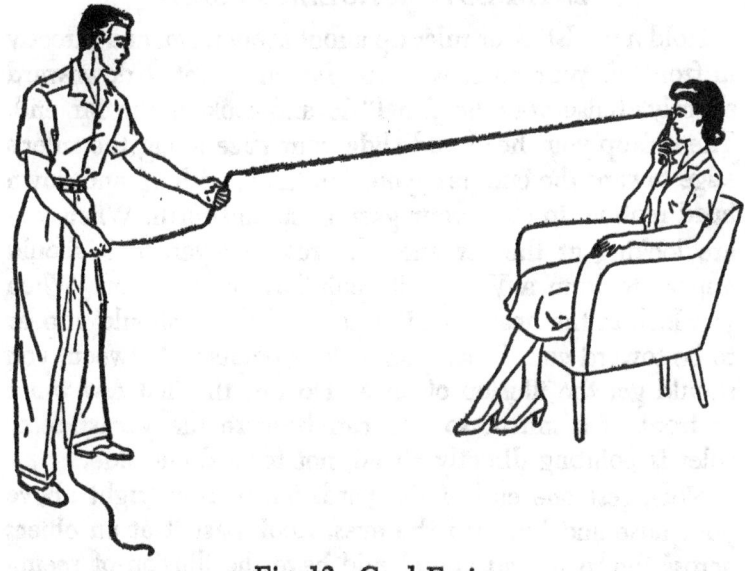

Fig. 12   Cord Fusion

Now ask your assistant to move the tube slowly—first a little closer to you and then farther away, no more than twelve to eighteen inches at a time. He should hold the tube with one hand and hold the cord taut with the other so that the cord forms a straight line, with no slack, as the tube is moved closer and farther away from you.

You should be able to converge, that is, to see the cord as a V, at distances ranging all the way from eight inches to twenty feet. When your convergence at all these points is good, then your fusion should be improved. Even though you can see the V perfectly, continue cord fusion practice while working with the other techniques to improve your sight.

If you work alone, start at the distance where you see the V and the X and gradually, over a period, move back until you lengthen the distance to twenty feet.

2. YARDSTICK-RULER FUSION

Hold a yardstick or ruler up a foot away from, and directly in front of, your nose, with the far end slanted downward slightly. Raise your head a little and look at the far end. Then, drop your head and slide your gaze along the ruler's edge toward the end near you. Continue, with up and down head motion, to slide your gaze back and forth. When you are looking at the far end, the ruler or yardstick should appear to form a V with its point away from you. When you look at the near end, the point of the V should appear to be toward you. When you look at points in between, you should get the illusion of an X. Do this the first few times in front of a mirror so you can be sure the yardstick or ruler is pointing directly ahead, not toward one side.

Now, rest one end of the yardstick or ruler right above your nose and between the eyes. Look past it at an object across the room and you should have the illusion of seeing the object in a channel formed by two yardsticks.

Even now, you can obtain some preliminary evidence of how important good fusion is in improving vision. For if you look at colored objects beyond the stick while practicing this technique, you will notice that the colors appear brighter. As you progress with the fusion techniques, letters, too, will appear brighter.

3. BOW FUSION

A child's toy bow, made of plastic, about ten inches long, purchasable at a dime store, has a cord which provides a fine edge for focus.

Use it as you used the yardstick or ruler. Slide your gaze

with a head motion along the cord, achieving the illusion of two cords forming a V. Then rest one end of the bow above the nose and look past the cord at an object across the room, again achieving the optical illusion of seeing the object in a channel formed now by two cords.

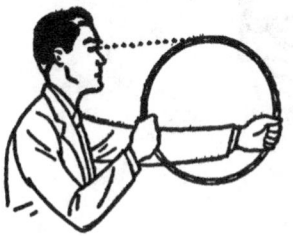 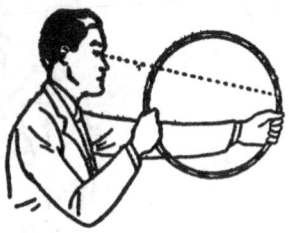

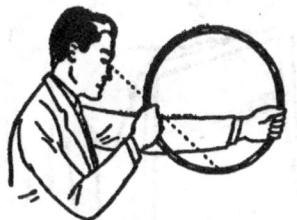

Fig. 13   Ring Fusion

4. RING FUSION

This technique is another step forward, introducing more distance accommodation and mobility into your fusion practice.

Use the same ring which you made for the ring-shifting drill in Chapter IV. Hold it a foot from, and directly in front of, your nose, with one edge of the ring toward you and the other away from you. (See Fig. 13.)

Now, with head motion, bring your gaze up the near side of the ring, over the top and down the inner edge of the far side. As you look at the near edge, it should be single while the far edge appears to be double. As you go down the far side, it should be single and the side toward you should appear to be double.

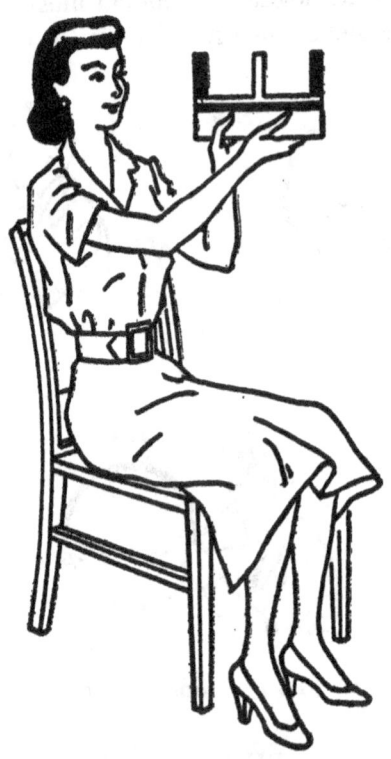

Fig. 14 Boat Fusion

Now come up your near side again, then raise the ring up to eye level and look past it at some object. The object will be single but the whole ring will appear to be double. The ring will be a channel through which you see the object.

5. BOAT FUSION

To make the simple equipment you'll need for this, get a piece of cardboard one foot long, eight inches high, and cut it out as shown in Fig. 14. The three projections represent boat masts. Using ordinary crayon, color one mast red on both sides, the second blue and the third yellow on both sides. A half-inch below the masts, running the length of the boat, draw a quarter-inch-wide line, and color it red on one side, yellow on the other. Make four of these boats—one twelve inches long, a second nine inches long, a third six inches long and the fourth two and a half inches. Cut them out all the same way and use the same colors.

Begin practice with the twelve-inch boat. Hold it up, slightly below eye level, directly in front of your nose, and out at a distance of at least eight inches from the tip of the nose. Now, raising and lowering your head, slide your gaze up and down the far mast. It should appear to be single, but both the middle and near masts should appear double. Next, with the same head motion, slide up and down the middle mast. Now, the middle mast should appear to be single, while the masts on both ends appear double. Look up and down the mast closest to you. It should now appear to be single while the other two masts appear to be double.

Now, finally look past all three masts at an object in the distance and you should be able to see a total of six masts with a red and a yellow line facing each other. You will get the sensation of looking down a channel between a set of three masts on one side and another set of three on the other. If you have difficulty, put the yellow line on the side of the weaker eye and have more light on that side.

6. PLATE FUSION

This technique is a further advance along the road to better sight since it helps achieve greater use of centralized vision along with better focusing and fusion.

On a file card, draw two circles, each the size of a dime, placed so their centers are two inches apart. Between them, draw a vertical red line a quarter-inch wide, from top to bottom of the card. Cut out the circles.

Hold the card up ten inches from your nose. The red line should be directly in front of your nose. (See Fig. 15.) Look through the two circles at an object across the room. You will get the illusion that you are viewing the object through a third hole centered between the two real ones and you should see a red line on each side of the imaginary hole.

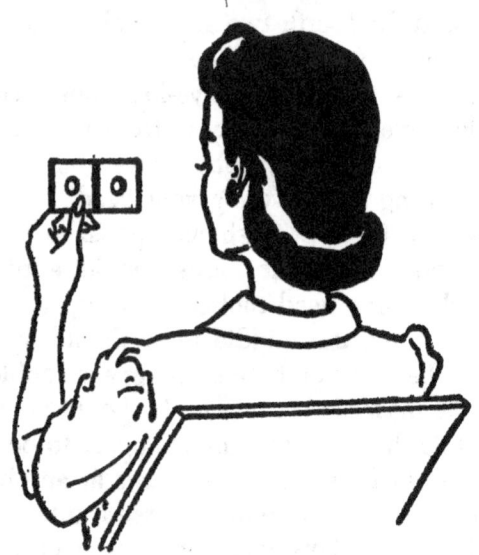

Fig. 15   Plate Fusion

7. CARD FUSION

Remember the check suggested at the beginning of this chapter? Did you try it and fail to merge the circles when you sighted along the yardstick? Now, after practice with the other techniques, you will be ready to accomplish the merging and help to perfect your fusion.

Draw the dime-size circles on a file card as suggested for the check—parallel to each other and one and one-half inches apart, with a vertical diameter in the left circle and a horizontal diameter in the right. For practice, too, make up other cards on which you can paste any two objects, letters, figures, designs, just so long as you have a pair of each, exact duplicates. The more cards you make up, the better for the sake of variety and interest.

On each card, paste the two duplicate objects parallel to each other with their centers one and a half inches apart. Between them, draw a vertical line, extending from top to bottom of the card.

Now, as with the original check, prop the card three feet away from you if you're nearsighted. Then raise a yardstick, with its narrow edge up, and place one end of it between your eyes and the other end on the vertical line of the card. If you're a farsight, substitute a ruler for the yardstick and hold the card at the end of the ruler.

Do the two objects now appear to merge into one and do you see the merged image in the channel between the two yardsticks or rulers?

If not, start a slight up and down head motion and you will see the images moving closer together until finally they merge. Looking beyond the end of the stick across the room and back to the card helps to merge images. It will help, too, to close your eyes and picture what the merged image should look like; then your mind will aid in the task of merging them. At first you will not be able to hold them merged for more than a second or so. But with continued practice, the image will stay fused.

You have seen how fusion can help make colors brighter. You will be able to apply the fusion techniques, too, to clearing letters and print. How to do this will be detailed in the next chapter.

Chapter VI

Accommodation: Learning to See Clearly at All Distances

Clear sight at all distances—vision that accommodates for near and far effectively and effortlessly—is your objective.

And now you are ready to begin gently and progressively to practice lengthening your vision if you are nearsighted, sharpening it at the near point if you are farsighted and equalizing vision in both eyes if one eye is weaker than the other.

You will not do it by making giant efforts. In the accommodation techniques that follow, you will be putting into use the elements of good vision you've learned about in preceding chapters. As you practice them, you will be substituting relaxation for tension, mobility for static looking, centralized vision with its use of the sharpest area of the retina in place of side sight and its use of the duller area, and good fusion with its effective use of both your eyes in place of disparate seeing. Your progress will be steady and pleasant, calling for no herculean straining and forcing. You will let good sight come to you rather than reach for it.

There are many techniques here. Some are useful in one type of vision loss but not in another. Many, however, are useful in all types of vision loss. There are enough for variety, and later, in the step-by-step chapter for your particular sight problem, you will find suggestions for which techniques to use one week and which another—for all need not be done simultaneously.

As you use these techniques, if you are nearsighted, you will be able to note and record progress, too. Vision is usually measured by doctors with testing charts at twenty feet, or with mirrored charts that provide a simulated twenty-foot distance. I as a teacher do not measure sight. You, however, can note your improvement in the following simple way. Keep track of your distance in terms of feet and inches. Each time you do one of these techniques a little farther away, if you are nearsighted, you show great improvement. If you are farsighted, each time you can read a smaller size of the graduated print in Chapter vm, you will have made a great gain.

Do not use trick vision in practicing these techniques or at any other time. Closing the eyes partially, popularly known as "squinting," may give you temporarily clearer vision but it is bad both for your sight and appearance. Other forms of trick vision, all of them harmful to good sight, include looking out the corners of the eyes, ducking the head and looking up, raising the head way up and looking way down.

Practice all of the techniques easily, naturally and without effort. Turn on the radio or record player and listen to music. The rhythm will help. And as you work remember what you have read about mobility and centralization. Keep your gaze and your head moving. Do not try to see everything at once.

In addition to practicing with both eyes together, you can and should do the drills with each eye separately, using an eye patch just as in working the mobility drills. Many eye tests, such as those given for driving licenses and in the armed services, require that one eye be covered. So this is good practice if you must take a test. But, more important, I have found that working the eyes separately often brings a rush of sight when the two are subsequently used together. Patching seems to speed up the return of good vision.

It also helps equalize vision if one eye is weaker. Work the weaker eye first. You'll be more patient, then, when you're fresher. Finishing with the stronger eye will take less time.

Another important point: Before switching a patch from one eye to another, always raise it and look around the room with both eyes before transferring it to the other eye.

It's also good policy, after working the eyes separately, to do one of the fusion techniques (Chapter v)—any one you choose.

1. JUMBLED NUMBERS

Fig. 16 shows a set of small jumbled numbers. You will need to make two more sets in larger sizes. They can be cut out from small and large calendars.

5	25	13	32	27	39
12	29	6	19	45	2
48	34	11	42	15	37
9	18	33	1	22	4
16	23	41	30	40	43
3	28	14	44	6	47
26	31	38	46	10	20
7	21	36	24	17	35

Fig. 16 Jumbled Numbers

Paste a set of each size on cardboards in the order shown. If you are nearsighted, hold this book at comfortable reading distance, open to Fig. 16. Place the intermediate-size set on a table or desk in front of you, far enough away so the numbers on it are a little blurred. Prop the large set out farther at a distance where they, too, are a little blurred.

Now, find the number 1 in Fig. 16, and pick out the 1's on the other two sets, proceeding from intermediate to large. Do the same with the numbers 2, 3, etc. Make your glances brief. No hunting is needed since the position of the numbers in all three sets is exactly the same. The whole purpose of the drill is to help establish the habit of shifting at various distances.

You can vary the drill for interest. For example, find the number 1 in Fig. 16, then the number 2 on the intermediate set and the number 3 on the far set, then come back to find 4 in Fig. 16, 5 on the intermediate set, 6 on the far set, etc.

Recently I have found it helpful to color the intermediate set with red water paint. I usually have my students do this after they have been retraining their vision for about six weeks. Although the red coloring somewhat obscures the intensity of the letters on the intermediate set, it seems to make it easier to see the far set.

If you are farsighted, place the largest set at a distance where every number is perfectly clear. Prop the intermediate set at a distance of four or five feet. Hold Fig. 16 at a distance where the numbers are slightly blurred. Proceed with the drill exactly as outlined above for the nearsighted, but work from the far set to the intermediate and then to Fig. 16.

After you've been working for six weeks or so, you will also find it helpful to color the intermediate set with red water paint.

2. JUMBLED LETTERS

Fig. 17 shows a jumbled letter set. You will need another set of larger size which you can make up with newspaper headline type. Use capital letters one-half to three-quarters of an inch high and lower-case letters about one-half the height of the capitals. Paste up the letters in the same order as in Fig. 17.

If you are nearsighted, place the larger set far enough away so the letters are a little blurred. Hold the set in the book at comfortable reading distance and find on it the little *a*. Then look out and find the big *A* on the distant set. Come back and find the little *b* on the book set, then look out and find the big *B* on the distant set. Continue through the alphabet.

O	g	Z	c	B	n	K	l
b	A	o	F	r	H	j	Y
U	k		t	C	a	Q	x
w	M	h	D	z	W	e	L
R		T	u	V	s		p
i	J	f	I		E	y	G
X	q	N	v	P	m	S	d

Fig. 17 Jumbled Letters

If you are farsighted, place the big set at a distance where it is clear and hold the book set at a distance where it is slightly blurred. Find the capital *A* on the distant set and then the small *a* in the book set and work through the whole alphabet.

3. PLAYING CARDS

This drill is helpful if you are nearsighted or wear bifocals and have lost distant sight. It is not for farsighted people.

Paste fifty-two playing cards on a large piece of cardboard. Mix the cards and arrange them in five rows—two top rows of eleven each and three bottom rows of ten each. Even better than pasting, attach the cards with photo-album "corners" so you can change the order if you find you are memorizing the card positions.

Place the board far enough away so the cards appear a little blurred. Sit down at a desk or card table with a duplicate deck. Shuffle and turn over the first card. If it is the ten of hearts, for example, look at the distant cards and find the ten of hearts. In doing so, don't stare, don't strain forward. Instead, begin at the left on the top row, slide your gaze with a head motion quickly across that row, then do the same in each succeeding row until you find the card. If it happens to be the second card from the left in the fourth row, place your hand card on the table in a similar position. Then, turn up the next card in the deck and proceed in the same fashion to find it on the distant set. Once again, place it on the table in a position corresponding to its location on the board. Work through the whole deck.

When your vision improves enough so that you can do this drill with the board out at a distance of six feet, you are ready to practice while wearing an eye patch. Work through one-half of the deck with the right eye covered, then finish the deck with the left eye covered. If one eye is considerably better in vision than the other, do more of the drill with the stronger eye patched and less with the weaker eye patched.

4. WATCH AND CLOCK

If you are nearsighted, glance at any number on your wrist watch and then at the corresponding number on a clock at a distance. Repeat with the other numbers. If you are farsighted, reverse the order—look from clock to watch.

This is a simple but valuable accommodation drill which you can practice many times a day—on the street, in an auditorium, theater or railroad station—anywhere you see a large clock. A few seconds of practice at a time will be helpful.

I had a cataract case in New York City who did this drill so much that he finally reached the point where he could see clearly the numbers on a big clock across the river in Edgewater, New Jersey, from his office in downtown New York.

5. MATCHING MAHJONG TILES, ADVERTISEMENTS AND OTHER MATERIAL

If you have a mahjong set, put a row of tiles on a table in front of you and place corresponding tiles in different order at a distance. If you are nearsighted, place the distant tiles out where they are a little blurred. If you are far-sighted, place them where they are clear and put the tiles in front of you at a distance where they are a little blurred. You may have to lean over to shorten the distance enough to make tiles blurred.

The object is to rearrange the tiles on the table into the same order as those at the distance.

You can do the same drill with material of any type that provides duplicate numbers, figures, letters or designs which you can match. You can even practice with two advertisements, both identical in layout, text and illustration, but of different size—perhaps an ad in *Time* and the same ad as it appears in *Life*. In the drill, simply find similar letters, numbers and designs in the far and near ads.

6. DOMINO WHEEL

Fig. 18 shows a domino wheel.

If you're farsighted, hold the wheel out at reading distance even though the dots are blurred. Go clockwise around the rim, with a head motion, and pick out all the "ones." Then, go counter-clockwise and pick out all the "twos." Go clockwise for "threes," counter-clockwise for "fours" and so on. As you work with speed and a head motion, the dots will become increasingly clear. Practice shifting your gaze up and down the vertical, horizontal and diagonal spokes, too. Don't try to count. Just be conscious of the white dots on the black background.

Another drill will help clear close point vision. Look at one of the "ones" in the hub, then quickly shift with a head

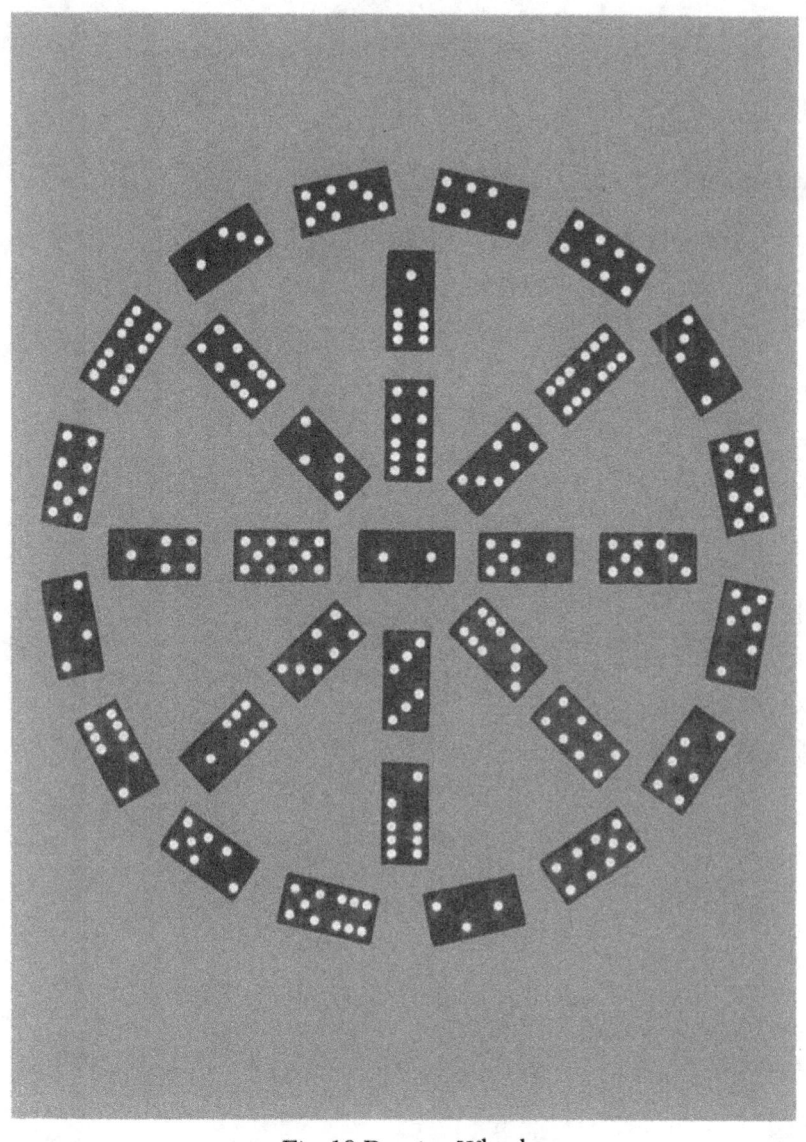

Fig. 18 Domino Wheel
(Also shown in color on inside front cover)

motion to one of the numbers in the rim. Go back to the number "one" in the hub and shift now, clockwise, to the next number in the rim. Work all the way around the rim.

If you're nearsighted, you will need a second, larger wheel. Buy a sheet of red poster board, sixteen inches square, usually available at any art supply or stationery store. You'll also need two sets of dominoes to paste up on the cardboard in the same order shown in Fig. 18.

Place the large wheel far enough away so the dominoes appear slightly blurred. Hold Fig. 18 at comfortable reading distance, look at the one-spot at the top of the vertical spoke of the wheel, then look out at the one-spot at the top of the vertical spoke on the distant wheel. Next look at the six-spot just underneath the one-spot on the nearer wheel and then at the six-spot on the far wheel. Proceed to work down the vertical spoke of the wheel; then pick some other spoke and go from one end of it to the other. Next day, you can work with two other spokes. The third day, you might start at the top of the wheel and work clockwise around the rim. The following day you might work counter-clockwise.

The domino wheel drill is a particularly helpful one for astigmatism. In astigmatism, there may be blurred vision. Light rays converge unequally in different meridians so that if you look at a wheel, the vertical spoke may be clear but the horizontal spoke blurred. After doing the domino wheel drill, the great majority of people with astigmatism whom I have taught have noted improvement.

7. LETTER BOARDS

This drill is one of the most valuable of all drills for improving distant vision.

Mr. E. L. Hurd of California has made a series of letter boards which our teachers use with nearsighted students. Each board has two sizes of letters.

You can make two boards of your own from the letters

printed at the end of this chapter. You can either cut them out or trace over them and duplicate them with black India ink.

Place the letters from the set marked "Letter Board 1" on a big piece of cardboard in four rows of twelve each, alternating large and small. Place those from set marked "Letter Board 2" on another piece of cardboard. It is better to put them on with photo-album "corners" rather than paste them on so you can change them when you are beginning to remember the order.

You will note also that there is a third set of letters called "Hand Tiles." Each of these should be pasted on a separate small piece of cardboard.

Begin work with board No. 1. Place it at a distance where the letters are slightly blurred. Seat yourself comfortably at a table on which you've placed the hand tiles. Pick up a letter, look at it briefly, then find the same letter on the distant board. Once you've found that, lay the hand tile down on the table in a position corresponding to its location on the distant board. Then pick up and glance at another letter and race your sight along the rows of letters on the distant board until you find it. Place this tile, too, in its proper position on the table. Continue working until you have finished all of the letters.

The letter board work can be done with one eye at a time, too. After working with one eye, rest briefly by sunning and palming. Then work the other eye and sun and palm again. The patch should be placed over the stronger eye first.

Use letter board No. 2, with its smaller letters, in the same way as No. 1.

Gradually, you will be able to work this drill with the boards farther and farther away. Measure the distance each time you practice so that you can keep records of your improvement.

You can use color to help speed progress. From time to

time, put a piece of yellow or red cellophane over the board so it covers all letters. Then do the first half of the drill with board covered, the remaining half with it uncovered. In doing the latter half, you will be able to move the board a little farther away and yet see the letters more clearly.

8. COMBINING FUSION WITH ACCOMMODATION PRACTICE

A great aid in helping to improve your accommodation both in the distance and at the close point is to use fusion techniques in conjunction with accommodation techniques.

Remember the yardstick-ruler fusion drill in Chapter v. As you rest one end of the yardstick above your nose, between the eyes, and look past it at an object across the room, you can achieve an optical illusion of seeing the object in a channel formed by two yardsticks, and if the object is colored, you notice that the color appears brighter.

Now you can apply this to clearing letters and print.

If you are nearsighted, when you have the letter board at a distance where the letters are blurred, channel with the yardstick, and through the channel you'll see the letters more clearly for a second. As you continue to practice fusion, accommodation and other techniques, the letters will begin to stay clear for longer periods. Later, they'll be clear without the channel.

If you are farsighted, use the same technique to help in clearing your near point vision. Working with a six-inch ruler, get your channel, then sight through it during your reading and other near point accommodation practice.

You can apply ring fusion, too, in accommodation practice. Use the ring to obtain a channel as described in Chapter v, then sight through it. If you are nearsighted, you can use the same ring you made for mobility and fusion practice. If you're farsighted, you will need to make a smaller ring for this. A shower curtain ring is good. Or you can form a circle, about silver dollar size, with a piece of black insulated wire. Wrap quarter-inch-wide pieces of white adhesive tape around your ring at intervals of a quarter of an inch.

In doing all the accommodation drills, remember to be relaxed. Occasionally stretch and yawn to help you relax. When you feel tired, stop and rest by sunning or palming, or both, and then go back, refreshed, to continue. Remember, too—and I repeat this because it is so important—to keep your gaze and head moving.

Your vision, as indicated earlier, will improve not by forcibly stretching it near or far, but rather by putting into use the basic habits of good vision.

You will be helped, too, in getting better and faster results with the accommodation techniques, by using along with them the mental aids you'll find in the next chapter.

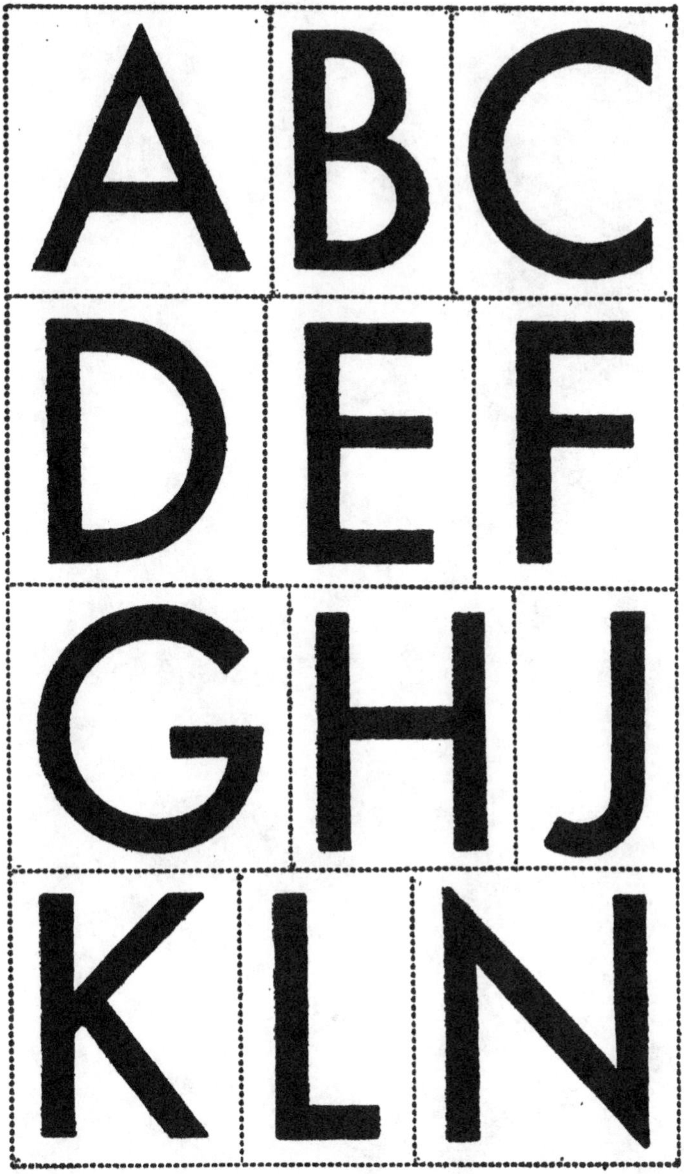

Fig. 19 Letterboard (1)

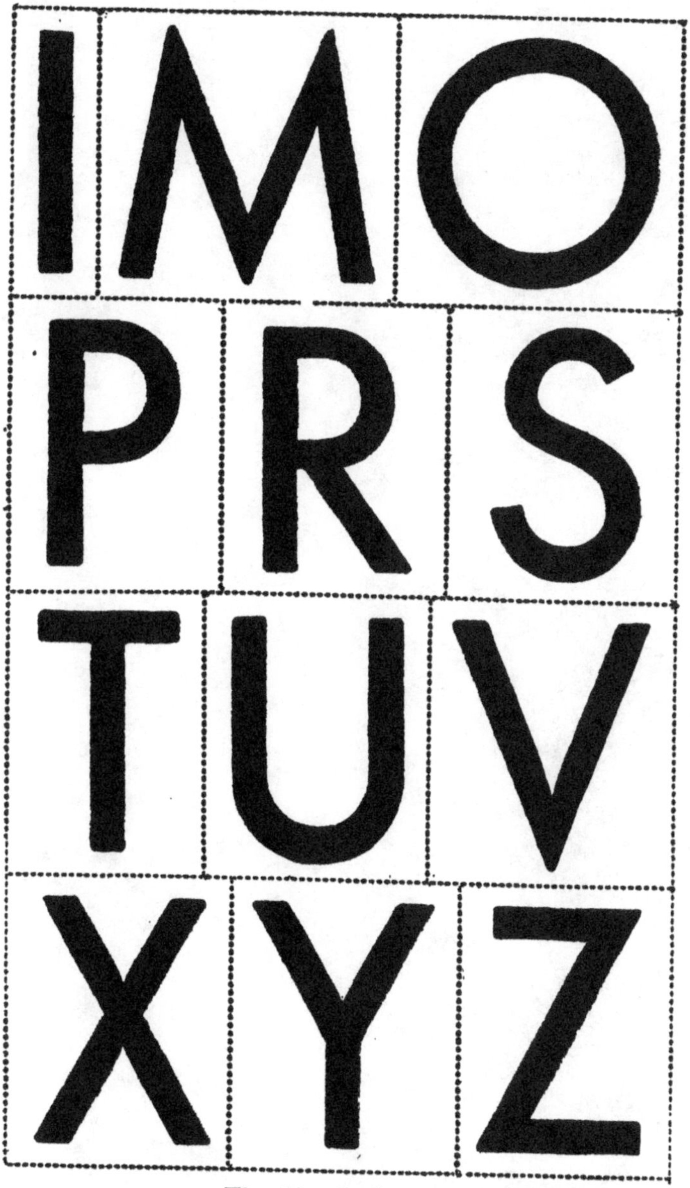

Fig. 19 *Continued*

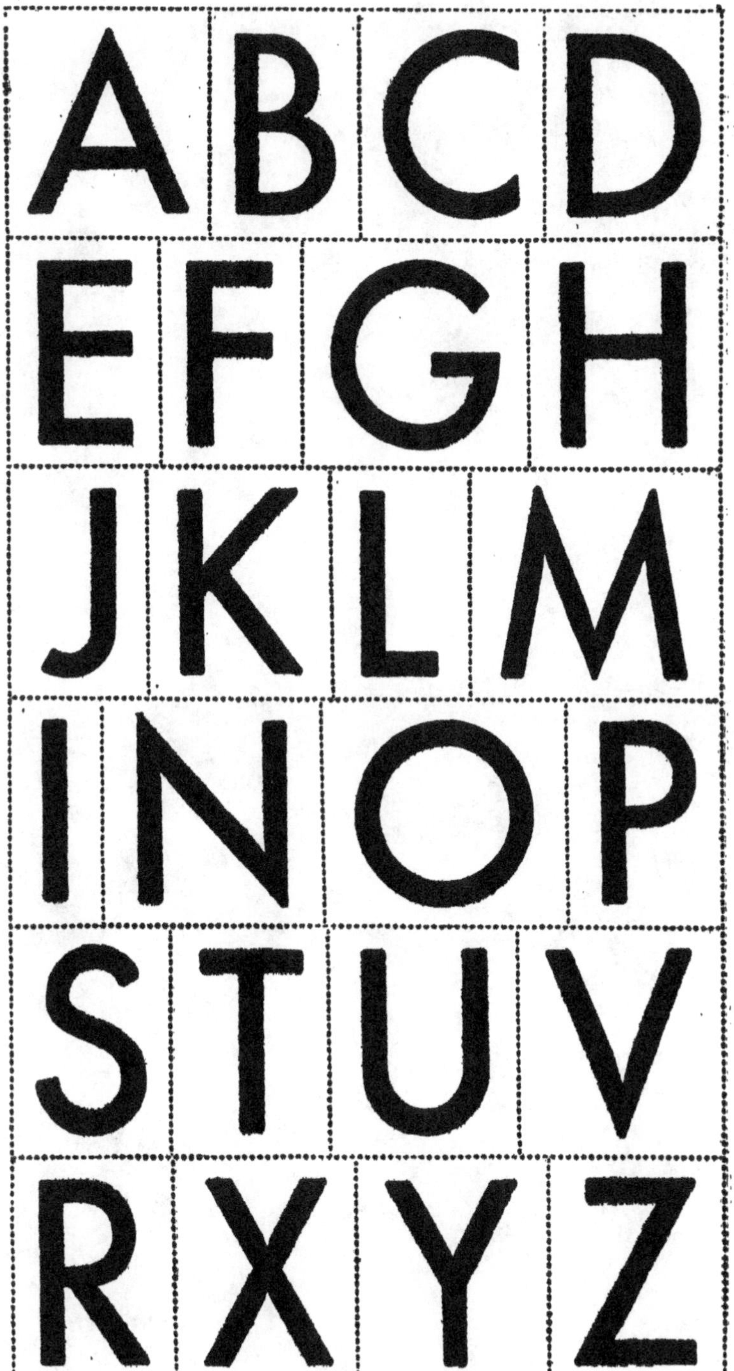

ABCD
EFGH
JKLM
INOP
STUV
RXYZ

Fig. 19 *Continued*

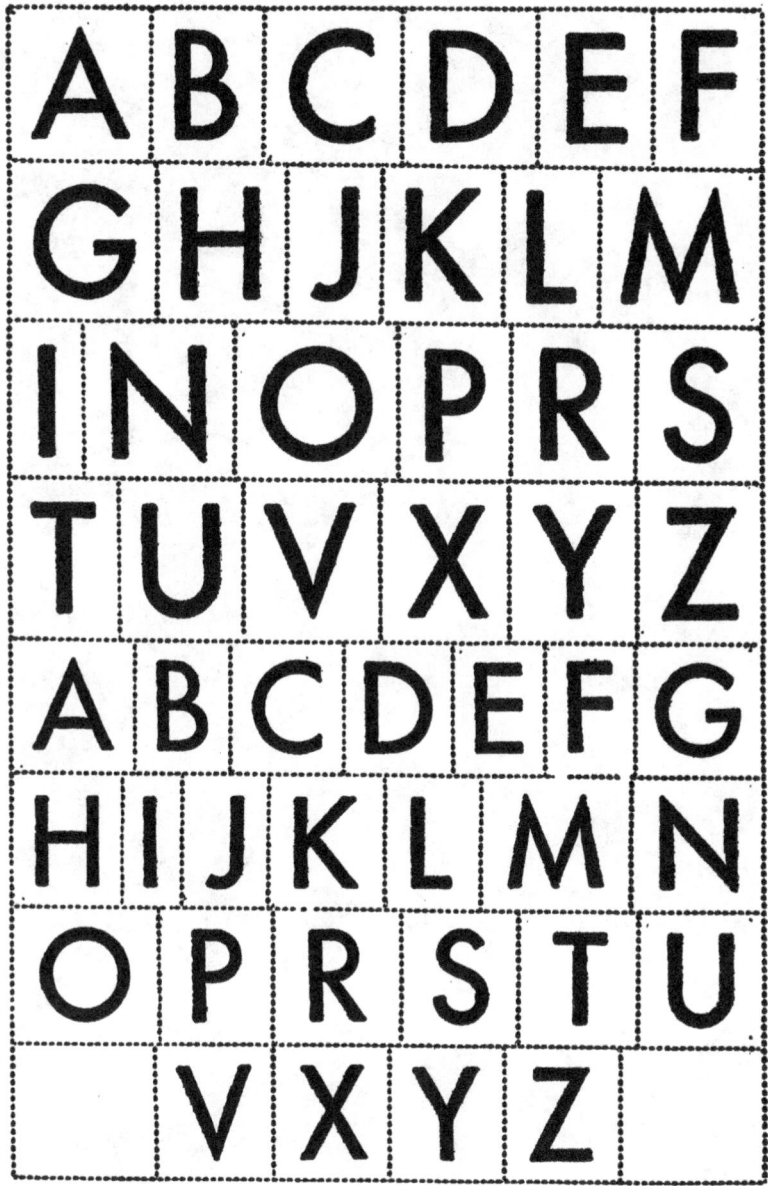

Fig. 20 Letterboard (2)

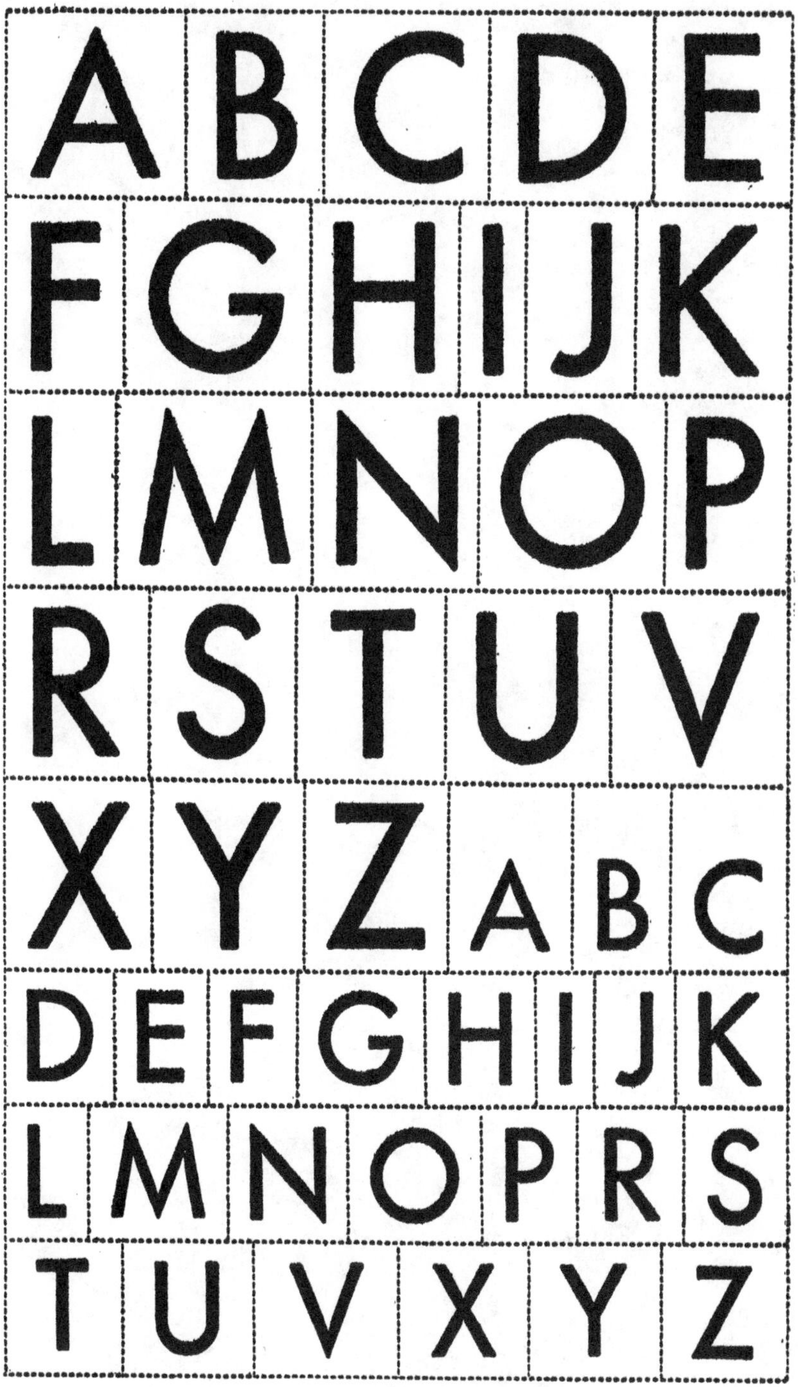

ABCDE
FGHIJK
LMNOP
RSTUV
XYZABC
DEFGHIJK
LMNOPRS
TUVXYZ

Fig. 21 Hand Tiles

Chapter VII

Mental Aids for Better Sight

No other organ of the body is so closely related to the mind as is the eye. Sight is at least as much psychological as physical—perhaps even more so.

The physical eye, like a camera or TV, transmits images. But it is in the mind that perception itself occurs. If you've ever been in a "brown study," you know that you can sit and stare at an object for an hour and, if your mind is otherwise occupied, it takes no note of what you are looking at. You do not perceive it then and you cannot recall it later.

Not only is the mind the end organ of sight; it also plays a role in controlling the functioning of the eye itself. For, as we have seen in Chapter II, once an image is picked up by the retina and transmitted to the brain, nerve impulses are flashed back from the brain to govern the action of the eye in focusing for distance and sharpening the image.

Whatever your sight problem, you will be helped to see better if you understand the role of the mind and make use of its powers to improve your sight.

After reading this chapter, you will be able to put certain specific mental aids to work in achieving further progress with the techniques given in previous chapters.

The first aspect of mental sight is curiosity. There seems to be a definite relationship between loss of curiosity and loss of sight. I have often found that the more the loss of sight, the less the curiosity to see. A nearsighted person with 20/30 vision will generally look around inquisitively

93

much more than one who has only 20/200 vision. A number of my students have been almost blind, their vision limited to object perception. Almost invariably, when they came to see me at my office, they stood in the doorway and expected to be led to a chair. Generally, on their first visit or two, I would oblige. Later, however, I would say, "Look around and you'll see the chair." As they would look around they would hesitantly call aloud such objects as cabinet, bookcase, pictures. Finally the exclamation would come: "Yes, I do see the chair!" It could just as well have been seen on a preceding visit—if there had been curiosity enough.

Loss of curiosity is often related to fear. After some loss of sight, many people, fearing they will not see well anyhow, lose curiosity to see. They do not make full use of the vision they have. And their vision, one might say, becomes rustier.

People with vision loss are often so convinced that they cannot see in some given situation or experience that they are virtually paralyzed into not seeing or even looking.

One psychiatrist has reported a number of nearsighted patients in his practice who were actually afraid to look at the stars at night—purely because of a fear that they would not be able to see distant objects.

A basic step in improving any vision loss is to develop curiosity. Begin to look inquisitively at all things around you. Start with those you can see clearly and go on to others that are hazy. The more curious you are, the more you put your sight to use as you practice improving your vision, the quicker your improvement will come. Counting and the other drills for increasing mobility and centralization given in Chapter IV help in this.

Mental sight also involves comparison and contrast. Your mind perceives by comparing and contrasting one thing against another. For example, psychological experiments have demonstrated that when you view a black object against a field of white, you actually see the black object by noting where the white touches it. In reading print, you note that an *H* differs from an *N* because the *H* has a square of white coming down from the top and another coming up from the bottom while the *N* has a wedge of white at both top and bottom.

You note that an *A* differs from an *X* because the *A* has white coming in from the base while *X* has white coming in from four sides.

Comparison and contrast help you identify round letters as you note that an *O* has no opening for white to come in, but a *U* has an opening at the top; the *C* has a wide opening at the right and *G* has less white at the right.

With normal sight, you make use of comparison and contrast automatically, unconsciously. Even with a sight loss, you make use of comparison and contrast at the distances at which you can see relatively well.

A conscious effort to make use of comparison and contrast for the next few months will be a great aid in helping you to learn to see better at distances at which you do not now see well.

For example, in my studio, when a nearsighted person works with the letter board, he may see the letter *R* in his hand but have difficulty in finding it in the distance. I have him slide his gaze along the rows of distant letters, thinking only of the letter *R*. If he mistakes the letter *B* for an *R*, I ask him to see if white comes in from the base. As he looks from white to white on each side of the letter, he sees the black line at the base of the *B*, and then continues his search for the letter R, now even more aware that he must find a letter which looks almost like a *B* except for that area of white coming in at the base.

In our work we constantly emphasize attention to background. For example, at virtually any distance, you will have no difficulty in seeing a piece of white cardboard, although you may have considerable difficulty in seeing the black letters on it. We ask our students to make no great effort to see or "pull in" letters, but rather to look first at the white on one side and then with a quick shift of the gaze to jump right over the letter to the white on the other side. It is amazing how, when they thus make no effort to pull in the black, it comes toward them and they see it more clearly.

Dr. Bates did a number of interesting experiments using a retinoscope, an instrument for determining the refractive state of the eye. With it he would measure the degree of nearsightedness in a patient who looked at an eye chart. When he made another measurement, this time with the chart turned over so that it was just a piece of blank white cardboard, the retinoscope would reveal that the eyeball was normal.

When farsights were examined while looking at a reading card at the close point, Dr. Bates reported the retinoscope revealed a high degree of farsightedness. But again, when the card was turned over so that the blank white side was revealed, the instrument showed a normal eye.

Make use of comparison and contrast when you practice the accommodation in Chapter VI. You will be helped, as already indicated, if you use contrast in picking out letters, distinguishing an *N* from an *H*, for example, by noticing where the white comes in.

You will be able to "clear" otherwise blurred images if you avoid staring and making great efforts to see them, and, instead, shift your attention from one area of white to another.

If your sight is very poor, you may have to begin by using a wide shift from white to white. Some farsighted people have to shift from one margin to another in a book held in the lap; some nearsighted people must begin with a shift from one edge to another edge of a letter board or jumbled number card. However, later, as vision gradually improves, the shifting can be narrowed. The farsight will get to the point of seeing clearly with a shift from front to back of a single word instead of from margin to margin of the whole book. The nearsight will be able to narrow down until he shifts from the white in front to the white behind a letter or figure.

The edging drill (Chapter IV) has already introduced you to the use of comparison and contrast.

As you continue to practice edging, you will get the optical illusion that the white at the edge of the object is a more intense white than the other areas of white. If you are farsighted, you will reach the point where a fast shift between two lines of print will seem to make the white between the lines lighter than other white areas on the page. And this will make the black seem blacker, which is an ultimate objective.

Memory is another vital aspect of mental sight.

Your mind's ability to interpret the images transmitted to it through the eye depends upon memory. You can see familiar objects much more clearly than those which are relatively strange. Evidently less energy is needed, too.

Some of my students have reported that, in their native New York, they can drive around for hours pointing out spots of interest to visitors without feeling fatigue, but when the tables are reversed, when they're being shown the sights of a strange city, they feel fatigued within an hour or two.

You can use memory to help your vision. Begin by improving your memory of letters and numbers. Close your eyes and try to see in your mind, one by one, the letters of the alphabet. Start with the letter A. Do you see it clearly both in upper and lower case? If you do not, open your eyes and look at the letters A and *a* on the jumbled letter card. Close your eyes again, and try to see them clearly now. When you've succeeded in this, go on to B and the other letters of the alphabet. You may be surprised to find that your memory of these basic building blocks of all knowledge is not as clear as you've thought.

As an interesting variation, start with the letter *I*. See it in your mind, then build from it all of the letters of the alphabet which use a straight line as part of their structure. Thus, for example, you can make the letter *B* by adding two loops to the straight line, and the letter *D* by adding a single half-circle. You can make the letter *E* by adding three arms.

As another variation, see in your mind all of the letters that are made up entirely of straight lines, such as *H*, *L* and *T*.

Go on to picture the letters that are entirely curved, like *C* and *O* and *S*. Then, picture those made of diagonal lines, such as *W*, *X* and *V*.

Any other little games you can devise to help improve your memory of letters, and numbers as well, will help.

The next step is to combine a memory of letters and numbers with a memory of seeing them more clearly in your mind at distances at which you do not see them clearly when your eyes are open. For example, if you are near-sighted and can see a particular size letter at a distance, let's say of eighteen inches, place the letter on a wall and look at it from eighteen inches away, then close your eyes, remember it, and with your eyes still closed try to visualize how the same letter would look at a distance of two feet instead of eighteen inches.

When you can see it clearly in your mind, step back to two feet, open your eyes and look at the actual letter on the wall. Look at it just for a split second. Then close your eyes again, picture how the letter would look at a distance of two feet, six inches, and when you can see it in your mind, take another half-step back, open and glance briefly at the letter on the wall and you will actually see it with your eyes.

When you do the accommodation drills given in Chapter VI, and encounter difficulty in seeing a letter clearly at a particular distance, close your eyes, remember the letter, see it clearly in your mind at that distance, then open your eyes and look at it.

If you are farsighted, hold a letter or word where you can see it clearly. Then close and visualize it perfectly two inches closer to you. When you can see it clearly in your mind, pull the letter two inches closer to you, open your eyes and look at it briefly. Continue doing this until you can bring it up to regular reading distance.

The same technique is of great value to people who are almost completely blind. Very frequently, I've found that the near blind have such great difficulty in mental visualization that it is necessary to begin by having them try to visualize their hand, often the last thing they saw before losing sight. Even then, to help them form a mental picture of the hand, it is often necessary to outline and tap their fingers. Once the hand can be pictured mentally, they soon begin to see it actually. And I have worked progressively forward from this to letters and numbers at distances, always proceeding first with the mental visualization and thereafter with the open-eye seeing.

Many people with great vision losses find it helpful to begin mental visualization with color, which they can often see in the mind when they cannot visualize letters or numbers. For example, if you can mentally picture green over a broad area, you can then proceed to trim the green area down to a point where you can visualize leaves on a tree or a green lampshade. Once you've done this, you can begin to visualize letters and numbers in color, then in black and white, and now you will begin to see them more clearly with eyes open.

I have noted this phenomenon, too, in many students—the ability to visualize most clearly those things remembered from the time when sight was perfect. Many students, unable to remember and describe objects in their own living room at home right now, can remember in great detail and with great clarity, objects in a room occupied as a child. It is sometimes helpful in the beginning to try to visualize these well-remembered objects from childhood or at any age when sight was good. Do not attempt, however, to visualize things to which unpleasant memories are attached. If anything, such memories will tend to reduce rather than increase vision.

Memory of things in motion is particularly valuable in improving sight. Close your eyes and visualize a speedboat darting across a lake, or a tennis game in which you follow, in your mind's eye, the flight of the ball back and forth across the net. Visualize a newsboy riding down a street, tossing papers up onto porches. If you visualize motion over a wide area, you will find that your head will move and you will also feel the movement of your eyes, even under the closed lids.

Eventually, you will be able to visualize in memory with your eyes open. For example, during the war, one pupil of mine who, while taking his Navy test, found the chart a little blurred looked above at the wall and visualized a white house in the distance clear across a wide lake. After that, he could drop his gaze and read the letters.

Another important aspect of mental sight is judgment. In looking at anything, after using contrast and comparison and memory, your mind must form a judgment about the object, an evaluation of what you've seen. You may evaluate it in terms of spatial relationship, shape, color and intensity of colors, motion and rhythm of motion. This is normal seeing.

Normal vision is lightning-fast. It is sight with speed achieved not by scrutinizing pauses but by quick glances aided by the mind and its lightning-fast analyses, evaluation and judgment.

If you are to read with ease and enjoyment, it will not

be by scrutinizing each letter but by fast glimpsing. And if in a quick glance you seem to see a word that begins with the letters Q and O, your judgment should almost instantly tell you that there is something wrong and that probably the second letter is not an O at all but more likely a U, since there is no word in the English language beginning QO.

If you're reading and come across a word that you think is "corn" but the word does not fit the context, your judgment will make you stop and take another look and you will probably think that the word is "earn," and, on the basis of this judgment, will actually be able to see the word "earn" more clearly.

You can depend on judgment to correct an error that speedy seeing may produce. It is also true that when you know through judgment what you *should* see, you are often able to see it better.

Actually, all of the mental aspects of sight take place almost simultaneously and are interactive. You cannot have judgment without memory, nor can you have contrast and comparison without curiosity. All work together.

That leads us into another phenomenon—the working together of the senses and how you can use other senses to aid sight.

Try this experiment if you are nearsighted. Place your jumbled letter card on a wall, then walk as far away from it as you can. Pick out a letter. If you cannot see it at all, walk toward it until you can at least faintly distinguish it as an O, for example, but stop at the point where it is still blurred. Now, close your eyes and imagine that you have just taken the first bite of some favorite food or delicacy. When you get an actual taste sensation, open your eyes and you will find that the O, for just a split second, will be clear. Now, close again and imagine you can hear a favorite sound —perhaps a song or orchestral work. When you can hear it in your mind, open your eyes and look at the letter, and again, for a split second, it will be perfectly clear. Close your eyes again and smell a favorite odor—perhaps the scent of a rose. Actually get a feeling that you are smelling the fragrance. Open your eyes again and once more, for a split second, the letter *O* will be perfectly clear.

You can do the same thing if you imagine that you are stroking the fur of your favorite pet, or running your fingers over a material that has a pleasant touch or a beautiful grain of wood.

Seeing is a mental function as well as a physical one.

Use the mental aids given in this chapter when you practice the accommodation drills described in Chapter VI. Use them, too, for the next few months, in all your seeing. They will help you to improve your sight more rapidly. You will make conscious use of them now—but later no conscious effort will be required. They will have become ingrained.

Chapter VIII

Reading Aids

If your vision at reading distance is poor, it will begin to improve as you practice the techniques already given. The additional aids presented in this chapter to be used in the reading practice sessions called for in your step-by-step program will add to and speed your improvement. They are specific aids designed to help you read with increasing ease and clarity.

When you practice reading and using these aids, leave your glasses off, of course. This may be a little difficult at first but you can start gradually, practicing only briefly in the first few days, gradually lengthening the sessions.

If your vision loss has been severe, at first, you may have to practice on large newspaper headlines. Gradually, you'll progress and be able to work with smaller subheads, then text.

Magazine advertisements are useful for reading practice because many contain various sizes of type.

In addition, some of your practice will be done with the special material in graduated print given at the end of this chapter.

Start working with the smallest size print you can read. Try to progress from there to the next smallest size. Your improvement and progress will not come by great leaps and bounds. It will come at first in little snatches of better sight, brief interludes when a letter or a word stands out clearly.

As you continue your practice, the flashes of good sight will lengthen until you consistently hold the gain.

1. BLINK AND BREATHE

Blink often as you read. Don't stare fixedly. And remember to breathe, regularly, easily. Watch for any tendency to try so hard and become so tense that you hold your breath as you read.

2. SUN AND PALM

Interrupt your reading frequently to sun and palm. Relaxation is a vital element in re-educating your vision. Don't rush and strain to get your practice done, to progress rapidly. Interruptions for sunning and palming are not "times out," but part of the practice and will speed your progress.

3. LOOK AWAY OFTEN

Stop reading from time to time to look away at something in the distance. Don't just raise your gaze without actually focusing on a distant object. Register its shape and color in your mind. When you return to the print, it will be a little clearer. If you're reading at night, the whole room should be illuminated, not just the area in which you are reading, so you can look up and see objects across the room.

4. SLIDE

Don't gobble your reading. In recent years, rapid reading has been stressed. Unfortunately, many people have learned to spread their sight as they read, covering several lines of print at a time. This habit may help you to read faster but not to see the print clearly.

You'll recall again that the fovea centralis, the area of clearest vision in the retina, can encompass only a small area—about a dime-size one at a reading distance of thirteen or fourteen inches. Trying to spread vision beyond that results in blurred vision.

Don't try to read in great snatches, seeking to take in whole lines at once and even several lines at a time.

Instead, slide your gaze along from margin to margin, keeping it mobile, using the fovea. Slide, not squarely on the line of print itself, but just underneath it—almost literally reading "between the lines." It may sound difficult, but isn't. You'll get it with a little practice. Sliding your gaze just under the line of print emphasizes the contrast between the print and the white space, and helps make the print appear to be blacker.

5. IMAGINE WHITENESS

Now and then close your eyes, and in your mind imagine a perfectly white sheet of paper. The print will appear blacker when you open your eyes again.

6. USE A WHITE PAPER

When print "grays out," cover the whole page of print with a piece of white paper. Imagine that you are drawing on it with white ink, a circle, square, triangle, or any other geometric figure. Slide the white paper off the printed page and now the print will seem much blacker.

7. USE A CARD OR SHIFTER

Place the edge of a file card just below the line of print. The extra whiteness provided by the card will make the line of print above it appear blacker.

Use the small red shifter. Run it back and forth with an inch shift—below the line of print—and it will help make the print clearer.

8. USE A RED PENCIL

Sharpen a red pencil to a fine red point. As you read, run the red point from one margin to the other directly under the line of print. Try to read the words as they appear over the top of the sliding pencil point. This will make the print seem brighter.

When a word is blurred, run the tip of the pencil back and forth underneath the word as you count its letters, and it will clear.

You can clear a blurred word, too, by jumping the pencil from the word in front to the one behind, back and forth several times.

9. SEE THROUGH A CHANNEL

Use the ruler technique as described in Chapter v. Look through the channel at the print held a few inches beyond the far end of the ruler. Within the channel, the words will briefly appear to be clearer.

10. SPEED READING

Some farsighted people read too slowly because the print is not clear enough to satisfy them. You will see the print more clearly by speeding your reading. Don't try to see many words at one time. Slide your gaze along—fast. For practice choose some light reading or, even better, something with which you are already familiar. Read as fast as you can, deliberately skipping words you don't see clearly. You'll see enough to get the meaning. As you continue to practice speed reading, there will be fewer and fewer words you do not see.

11. PRACTICE WITH COLOR

This is helpful in learning to read poor print and poorly lighted print when it's essential to do so. You'll need an old magazine such as *Reader's Digest*. Leave the first page white. Paint the second with a pale yellow water color. Leave the third page white and color the fourth page pale green. Skipping another page, color page 6 red. Color page

8 pale blue. Continue this order of coloring throughout the first half of the magazine.

Occasionally, in your daily practice, use the magazine for ten minutes or so at a time. As you read the alternate white and colored pages, you will be accustoming your sight to reading difficult material. Print on white background will then seem easy.

12. USE A TINY-PRINT BOOKMARK

If you can find tiny print—perhaps, in an old book or the back of a bill of lading—cut out strips that you can use as bookmarks. Then, even in your casual reading, whenever print begins to blur, read the tiny print on the bookmark. The latter may be blurred, too, but your sight will pick up when you go back to regular print.

13. PATCH AND READ

You will also be helped in building your reading ability by working with each eye separately, patching the unused eye. Many people have a stronger eye on which they may put most of the burden of reading. Practice with each eye separately will help to build up equal vision in both eyes.

Place the patch over the stronger eye, then read with the weaker eye. At first read for a very short period, perhaps only five minutes. Always remember to stop *before* you become tired.

Take your patch off and look around the room with both eyes. Then place the patch over the weaker eye and read for a short period of time with the stronger one.

It is important to remember to hold the print *in front of the eye patch* so that when you read with one eye you are looking slightly inward. (See Fig. 22.)

After patching, you will find that you will get greater clarity and speed with the two eyes together.

All of these techniques will be of great value in building

up your reading vision. Use them in the reading practice sessions called for in your step-by-step program given in a later chapter.

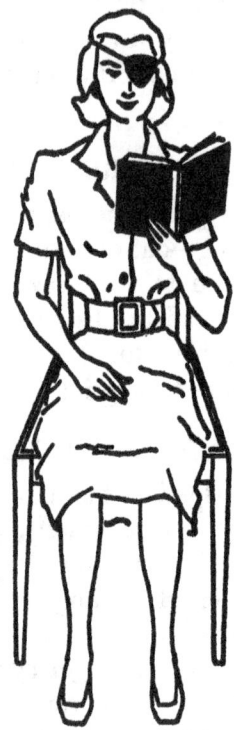

Fig. 22   Reading with a Patch

They may seem artificial and, of course, in themselves, they are. They're designed to be practice aids which will help establish proper vision habits, and the more you apply them in practice, the sooner the habits will take hold and conscious use of the aids will become unnecessary.

Mental Sight

1. Sight is mind and eye coordination. It is more mental than physical.

2. The eye sees but the mind must interpret and evaluate what is seen.

3. There are five basic components of mental sight: curiosity, contrast, comparison, memory and judgment.

4. Curiosity means intelligent visual searching, that is, looking around just as if you saw everything with perfect clarity.

5. Counting objects and colors is the best way to achieve curiosity.

6. Contrast is the gradations of difference in foreground and background.

7. For instance, the print on this card will appear blacker if you will close your eyes for a moment and imagine clearly a sheet of clean, white paper before opening them again.

8. Comparison is the evaluation of similarity and difference. A capital "H" and a capital "N" both have two parallel sides; but the "H" has a horizontal bar, while the "N" has a diagonal line.

9. Memory is the sum total of our learned and our recollected experiences.

10. Judgment is the summation, the end result, the interpretation or evaluation of what the eye sees.

11. These mental activities should be simultaneous and interrelated.

12. Perfect sight means perfect mental coordination.

Fig. 23   Mental Sight

Seattle

1. Seattle is the largest city in the State of Washington.

2. Like Rome it covers seven hills.

3. Often called "The Gateway to Alaska" it has retained some of the carefree manner of a frontier town.

4. Its docks are redolent of its trade with Alaska and the Orient. Seattle's harbor is also one of the commercial fishing centers of the world.

5. The industries of Seattle range from wood furniture factories and chemical laboratories to the sprawling Boeing plant where the great bombers are built.

6. The University of Washington, inside the city limits of Seattle, has a campus that is considered one of the largest and most beautiful in the world.

7. Because of Washington's tremendous interest in the lumbering and fishing industries, the University maintains large forests and biological laboratories far from the campus.

8. Most of the atomic research done on fish is centered at the University.

9. From Seattle's downtown streets you can smell salt air from the bay and by looking down the streets you can catch glimpses of the great mountains of the Olympic and Cascade Ranges.

10. The proximity of the bay, Lake Washington and smaller lakes makes it possible for almost everyone to build his home where he has a view of both water and mountains.

11. Its climate is mild. Seattle gardeners may grow roses the year around. Like Ireland, the countryside is always green and the water always blue.

12. It is a beautiful city set in emerald and turquoise.

Fig. 24 Seattle

Fourscore and seven years ago our fathers brought forth upon this continent a new nation, conceived in liberty and dedicated to the proposition that all men are created equal. Now we are engaged in a great civil war, testing whether that nation, or any nation so conceived and so dedicated can long endure. We are met on a great battlefield of that war. We have come to dedicate

Fig. 25 Gettysburg Address (1)

Fourscore and seven years ago our fathers brought forth upon this continent a new nation, conceived in liberty and dedicated to the proposition that all men are created equal. Now we are engaged in a great civil war, testing whether that nation, or any nation so conceived and so dedicated can long endure. We are met on a great battlefield of that war. We have come to dedicate a portion of that field, as a final resting-place of those who here gave their lives that that nation might live. It is altogether fitting and proper that we should do this. But in a larger sense we cannot dedicate, we cannot consecrate, we cannot hallow, this ground. The brave men, living and dead, who struggled here, have consecrated it, far above our poor power to add or detract. The world will little note,

Fig. 26 Gettysburg Address (2)

Fourscore and seven years ago our fathers brought forth upon this continent a new nation, conceived in liberty and dedicated to the proposition that all men are created equal. Now we are engaged in a great civil war, testing whether that nation, or any nation so conceived and so dedicated can long endure. We are met on a great battlefield of that war. We have come to dedicate a portion of that field, as a final resting-place of those who here gave their lives that that nation might live. It is altogether fitting and proper that we should do this. But in a larger sense we cannot dedicate, we cannot consecrate, we cannot hallow, this ground. The brave men, living and dead, who struggled here, have consecrated it, far above our poor power to add or detract. The world will little note, nor long remember, what we say here, but it can never forget what they did here. It is for us, the living, rather to be dedicated here to the unfinished work which they who fought here have thus far so nobly

Fig. 27 Gettysburg Address (3)

Fourscore and seven years ago our fathers brought forth upon this continent a new nation, conceived in liberty and dedicated to the proposition that all men are created equal. Now we are engaged in a great civil war, testing whether that nation, or any nation so conceived and so dedicated can long endure. We are met on a great battlefield of that war. We have come to dedicate a portion of that field, as a final resting-place of those who here gave their lives that that nation might live. It is altogether fitting and proper that we should do this. But in a larger sense we cannot dedicate, we cannot consecrate, we cannot hallow, this ground. The brave men, living and dead, who struggled here, have consecrated it, far above our poor power to add or detract. The world will little note, nor long remember, what we say here, but it can never forget what they did here. It is for us, the living, rather to be dedicated here to the unfinished work which they who fought here have thus far so nobly advanced. It is rather for us to be here dedicated to the great task remaining before us; that from these honored dead we take increased devotion to that cause for which they here gave the last full measure of devotion; that we may here highly resolve that these dead shall not have died in vain; that this nation under God, shall have a

Fig. 28   Gettysburg Address (4)

Fourscore and seven years ago our fathers brought forth upon this continent a new nation, conceived in liberty and dedicated to the proposition that all men are created equal. Now we are engaged in a great civil war, testing whether that nation, or any nation so conceived and so dedicated can long endure. We are met on a great battlefield of that war. We have come to dedicate a portion of that field, as a final resting-place of those who here gave their lives that that nation might live. It is altogether fitting and proper that we should do this. But in a larger sense we cannot dedicate, we cannot consecrate, we cannot hallow, this ground. The brave men, living and dead, who struggled here, have consecrated it, far above our poor power to add or detract. The world will little note, nor long remember, what we say here, but it can never forget what they

Fig. 29 Gettysburg Address (5)

Fourscore and seven years ago our fathers brought forth upon this continent a new nation, conceived in liberty and dedicated to the proposition that all men are created equal. Now we are engaged in a great civil war, testing whether that nation, or any nation so conceived and so dedicated can long endure. We are met on a great battlefield of that war. We have come to dedicate a portion of that field, as a final resting-place of those who here gave their lives that that nation might live. It is altogether fitting and proper that we should do this. But in a larger sense we cannot dedicate, we cannot consecrate, we cannot hallow, this ground. The brave men, living and dead, who struggled here, have consecrated it, far above our poor power to add or detract. The world will little note, nor long remember, what we say here, but it can never forget what they did here. It is for us, the living, rather to be dedicated here to the unfinished work which they who fought here have thus far so nobly advanced. It is rather for us to be here dedicated to the great task remaining before us; that from these honored dead we take increased devotion to that cause for which they here gave the last full measure of devotion; that we may here highly resolve that these dead

Fig. 30 Gettysburg Address (6)

Fourscore and seven years ago our fathers brought forth upon this continent a new nation, conceived in liberty and dedicated to the proposition that all men are created equal. Now we are engaged in a great civil war, testing whether that nation, or any nation so conceived and so dedicated can long endure. We are met on a great battlefield of that war. We have come to dedicate a portion of that field, as a final resting-place of those who here gave their lives that that nation might live. It is altogether fitting and proper that we should do his. But in a larger sense we cannot dedicate, we cannot consecrate, we cannot hallow, this ground. The brave men, living and dead, who struggled here, have con-

Fig. 31 Gettysburg Address (7)

Fourscore and seven years ago our fathers brought forth upon this continent a new nation, conceived in liberty and dedicated to the proposition that all men are created equal. Now we are engaged in a great civil war, testing whether that nation, or any nation so conceived and so dedicated can long endure. We are met on a great battlefield of that war. We have come to dedicate a portion of that field, as a final resting-place of those who here gave their lives that that nation might live. It is altogether fitting and proper that we should do this. But in a larger sense we cannot dedicate, we cannot consecrate, we cannot hallow, this ground. The brave men, living and dead, who struggled here, have consecrated it, far above our poor power to add or detract. The world will little note, nor long

Fig. 32 Gettysburg Address (8)

Fourscore and seven years ago our fathers brought forth upon this continent a new nation, conceived in liberty and dedicated to the proposition that all men are created equal. Now we are engaged in a great civil war, testing whether that nation, or any nation so conceived and so dedicated can long endure. We are met on a great battlefield of that war. We have come to dedicate a portion of that field, as a final resting-place of those who here gave their lives that that nation might live. It is altogether fitting and proper that we should do this. But in a larger sense we cannot dedicate, we cannot consecrate, we cannot hallow, this ground. The brave men, living and dead, who struggled here, have consecrated it, far above our poor power to add or detract. The world will little note, nor long remember, what we say here, but it can never forget what they did here. It is for us, the living, rather to be dedicated here to the unfinished work which they who fought here have thus far so nobly advanced. It is rather for us to be here dedicated to the great task remaining before us; that from these honored dead we take increased devotion to that cause for which they here gave the last full measure of devotion; that we may here

Fig. 33 Gettysburg Address (9)

Fourscore and seven years ago our fathers brought forth upon this continent a new nation, conceived in liberty and dedicated to the proposition that all men are created equal. Now we are engaged in a great civil war, testing whether that nation, or any nation so conceived and so dedicated can long endure. We are met on a great battlefield of that war. We have come to dedicate a portion of that field, as a final resting-place of those who here gave their lives that that nation might live. It is altogether fitting and proper that we should do this. But in a larger sense we cannot dedicate, we cannot consecrate, we cannot hallow, this ground. The brave men, living and dead, who struggled here, have consecrated it, far above our poor power to add or detract. The world will little note, nor long remember, what we say here, but it can never forget what they did here. It is for us, the living, rather to be dedicated here to the unfinished work which they who fought here have thus far so nobly advanced. It is rather for us to be here dedicated to the great task remaining before us; that from these honored dead we take increased devotion to that cause for which they here gave the last full measure of devotion; that we may here highly resolve that these dead shall not have died in vain; that this nation under God, shall have a new birth of freedom, and that government of the people, by the people, for the people, shall not perish from the earth.

Fig. 34 Gettysburg Address (10)

Chapter IX

All Day Long

One of the happiest aspects of improving your vision is that it need not be a burdensome process—a chore for which you must set aside hours every day.

You have now seen all the basic techniques that have proved useful in overcoming various types of vision loss. A selection of those which you will use for your particular problem—along with modifications to increase their value for you—will be presented in a later chapter which will also guide you on when to practice them, in what order and for how long.

Each day, you'll need only an hour or so for formal drilling. You will need even less, and your progress will be faster, if you take advantage of opportunities all day long for informal practice. You can practice casually on many occasions for just a minute or even a few seconds at a time. The practice can be a restful *divertissement*. And it is just such casual practice, integrating the techniques of good vision into the whole fabric of your daily life, which gives you a firmer grip on them and converts techniques you have to think about into good habits of seeing that require no conscious effort.

Is it a sunny day? Go to a window now and then and take the sunlight on your closed lids. Do this several times even if for no more than thirty seconds at a time, and you will be helping your sight to a valuable extent. You'll find it practical, on many occasions, to sun briefly while riding on a bus or train. More than practical, you'll find it desirable and be

117

eager to seize opportunities after you note the results. And this applies to all the other methods of helping your vision.

Palming during the day? If you're an executive or a housewife, anyone who has some privacy, there will be many times when you can palm for a minute or two. If you have little or no privacy at work, if you're a desk worker in a busy open office, for example, you can still find opportunities. Are there times when, a little tired by the job, you take a minute or two to sit idly at your desk with your head in your hands, trying to recuperate? Instead, palm for a minute or two. If you'd like to make your palming more unobtrusive, you can palm one eye at a time. If you can do no more, it's relaxing and beneficial to close your eyes and just imagine that you are palming.

Whatever your occupation, there are probably at least a few times during the day when you have a moment or two of enough privacy to do a few long and short swings.

When walking to and from work, you can practice swinging by looking from a sign or a store window or anything at all on the opposite side of the street over to something on your side of the street, at least twenty feet in front of you.

Practice deeper breathing. Many people tend to breathe too shallowly, some tend even to hold the breath when trying to see something. The reverse is helpful.

When you're walking, breathe in as you take four steps, breathe out as you take another four steps. Think: "In-two-three-four, out-two-three-four," and keep in step to that rhythm. You can also achieve rhythmic breathing while walking if you hum a lilting tune silently to yourself. When you're seated now and then make a point of doing this: First, let all the air out of your lungs and then breathe in and hold the breath for a few seconds and go on to breathe in some more, adding to the first breath. Let all the air out and do it once more. You'll find this especially helpful when you're feeling tense. It tends to relax the whole body as well as to improve vision.

Any time you can substitute relaxed habits for tension-producing ones, you help your sight—as well as your whole body.

Do you stand stiffly on both feet when waiting for a bus, your body tense and your eyes staring? Instead, shift from one foot to the other and you'll feel more relaxed and there will be less tendency to stare.

Unless you are physically incapacitated, or extremely near-sighted, drop a pencil or any small object now and then and bend over to pick it up. The change in posture helps to relieve muscular tension, improve circulation and promote relaxation.

You can find many opportunities for improving mobility and centralization. If you're a man, shave without your glasses and follow the movement of your razor in the mirror. Follow your hand movements as you knot your tie and comb your hair.

If you're a woman, watch in the mirror as you apply lipstick and comb your hair. When you go through your closet looking for something to wear, swing your gaze back and forth across the lineup of apparel.

At breakfast and all other meals, watch the movements of your spoon as you stir your coffee. Observe the texture, color and shape of the food. Look back and forth a few times from knife to fork. With a circular head motion edge the rim of a plate.

Do you "doodle" when you're on the telephone? A good way to get practice in mobility is to watch the point of your pencil. Now and then, too, pick up a pencil and edge it. And on your way to and from work, take a moment to stop and look in a window and count the objects with touches of a particular color.

Anything which makes you break your stare—edging or counting objects, watching movement of any kind—is a help in achieving mobility and centralization.

Practice mobility, centralization and relaxation, especially after your day's work is done. On your way home, count some objects, edge a few others, shift your gaze, do a little deep breathing. You'll feel less tired, more relaxed when you arrive, and you'll enjoy your dinner and the whole evening more.

How can you practice fusion during the day? If you're a smoker light your cigarette and then move the lighted match out six to eight inches in front of your nose. Look past it at an object across the room. The match flame will appear to be double.

While you're smoking, hold your cigarette up occasionally so the ashes are at the top. If you hold it at a distance of six to eight inches from your nose and look past it at an object across the room, you will see two lighted ends and two spirals of smoke.

When you ride a bus, try to get a seat in back of one of the stanchions. Look up and down the stanchion then beyond it, and the stanchion will appear to be double.

As you sit at your desk, hold a pencil out horizontally with the pointed end away from you and nine or ten inches from your nose. Raise your head and look out at the point of the pencil. It will appear to be single and the eraser will appear to be double. Drop your head and let your gaze rest briefly halfway between the point and the eraser. That particular spot will appear to be single but now you will seem to see two points and two erasers—in effect, an X. Drop your head still farther and look at the eraser which now will appear to be single while the point will appear to be double. Occasionally look past the pencil at an object in the distance, and you will have an illusion of a channel made of two pencils.

Shifting focus from near to far can also be practiced many times during the day. When you're walking down a street, look down at the line in the pavement, then follow it out in the distance with a head motion. When you come to a corner, glance down at the near curb, then across the street to the far curb. If you're carrying a handbag or a package, look at one edge, then look at the edge of a sign or building in the distance.

If you're walking down the street and see a large clock in the distance, seize the opportunity to look at your wrist watch and compare the time.

When you're riding in a bus or car, glance down at your newspaper, pick out a letter, then look off to the distance and see if you can find a sign with a similar letter.

On a bus, look at the advertising signs and pick out the alphabet, one letter at a time. Find some of the letters on street signs. If you're at the rear of a bus, look from ear to ear of the people sitting in front of you, then up to the back of the driver's head. And from there, go on to look out to the road ahead.

In all of this work, you're aiming to improve accommodation—your ability to see with clarity at near and far points. Anything you do to shift your gaze from a near object to a far one, or vice versa, with brief little glances and always with head motion, is excellent for the purpose.

One important help, especially for nearsighted people: If you look at an object in the distance and are unable to see it clearly, try looking beyond to something still farther away. Never mind whether you can see the more distant object clearly. When you bring your gaze back to the closer original object, you will find that it has become a little clearer.

In my office in Seattle, while working with nearsights who wanted to get into the armed forces, I often asked a boy who was having trouble seeing at twenty feet to look out the window across the harbor of Seattle, to the outline of West Seattle hill, two miles away. When he turned back to the letters, he could see them more easily.

The more creative you are in devising ways in which you can practice all the good visual techniques, the better the results you will achieve—and the faster.

. I have found it helpful to encourage my students to make little job analyses—to study their daily schedule in order to find all the periods and activities during which it would be feasible to go without glasses and to do some practicing.

Perhaps you'd like to try to analyze your daily schedule.

Sit down with pencil and paper and go through an average day in your life, from the moment you wake up in the morning until the moment that you go to bed at night.

List, in chronological order, all your activities. Are you, for example, serving or eating breakfast at eight? Riding a bus or train at 8:30? Taking a coffee break at ten? Driving a car at eleven? Making beds at 11:30? Right down the line, what are the various activities you're engaged in at all times of the day?

Opposite the items on your list, indicate those in which, even if for no more than a minute at a time, you might go without your glasses and do a relaxation drill, a mobility drill, a fusion drill, or an accommodation drill.

You can count on being surprised at the total time you can put to use for practice time.

Let's suppose you're having lunch at home. Could you eat without your glasses? And could you have the large domino wheel hung up on the wall across the room, and the small domino wheel at the table? And could you, at this point, get in a minute or two of the domino wheel practice?

If you are a business executive, could you take off your glasses now and then when you dictate and look down at a paper in your hand and then look out the window?

If you are a nearsighted secretary, could you for at least part of dictation time take off your glasses, even if you must hold your pad closer to you, and glance up now and then from your notebook to the person dictating or even, on occasion, out the window and back again?

If you're a high-school or college student, could you take off your glasses while changing classes and look down to the books you're carrying under your arm, and then quickly away and down the length of the corridor? Could you count people in the corridor and the books under their arms, or edge a water faucet as you pass? If you're listening to a lecture, could you take notes without glasses—and look from the point of your pencil to the lecturer and then back again? If you stare idly around, as most students do on occasion during a lecture, could you look purposefully around, counting objects and colors in the room, edging the ears of the person in front of you, or pictures on the wall?

The job analysis is really a simple but valuable device. By analyzing your typical day, you'll discover how much time there is to be used for practice in improving your vision. Moreover, the analysis has another value. The drills you will use fall into four classifications—relaxation, mobility and centralization, fusion and accommodation. The objective is to get a maximum amount of drilling under each classification each day. The job analysis will help you to plan for this.

Improved vision comes when you use your eyes and mind properly—when poor habits are discarded and replaced by good ones.

Casual practice all day long will greatly speed your progress.

Chapter X

In Games and Fun

Leisure-time activities can be used to increase your sight. You can literally practice with fun. You can count the time spent watching television or movies as part, and a most helpful part, of your practice. You can speed up your sight improvement as you motor, watch or engage in sports, view movies and TV, play card and other games.

The suggestions that follow will help you do this as they have helped people with many types of vision difficulties. In all leisure-time activities, you will actually improve your sight only when your glasses are off. But you need take them off only for brief periods at first. Gradually, you will be able to keep them off longer and longer in comfort—and with better and better results.

MOTION PICTURES

Ever since the first flickering nickelodeon, the movies have had a reputation for causing headaches and strained vision. However, many of the people connected with the movie industry who are required to see hundreds of pictures a year have excellent sight. Watch one of them and you will see that in viewing a movie, he uses naturally the techniques that maintain good vision. He changes focus, shifts, keeps his sight mobile.

Mobility, as we've seen earlier, is a fundamental of good sight. It can be increased by watching objects in motion, and movies provide an excellent opportunity.

When you look at movies, keep shifting your vision. Don't try to see everything on the screen at once but rather, look rapidly from one person or object to another. If a large close-up is shown, trace around head and face.

Blink your eyes at a normal rate, and look away now and then from the screen.

Now and then turn your head slowly to one side and look at the face of someone sitting nearby or count the exit signs around the theater. All of this shifting is of such short duration that you will not lose the continuity of the story.

Don't lower your head and look up at the screen. This is unnatural focus for the eyes, unnatural position for the head. Tilt your head up or down, depending upon where you sit, so your nose is pointing at the screen.

If you're nearsighted, you can improve your distant vision by watching movies. Begin by keeping your glasses off for short periods and by sitting as close to the screen as necessary, perhaps first-row orchestra. Gradually, you will be able to sit farther and farther back and to go without your glasses for longer periods. Eventually, you may be able to view an entire movie comfortably and clearly without glasses and at the back of the theater.

If you are farsighted, you can use movies to help your close point vision. Start by viewing a movie for a short period without glasses while seated at the back or middle of the theater. Gradually move forward. As you become able to sit closer and closer, you'll find a steady improvement in your reading vision.

If you're cross-eyed, you can help to straighten your eyes by sitting to the side of the theater. If your right eye is turned in, or the left eye is turned out, sit on the left side of the house. If the left eye is turned in, or the right eye turned out, sit on the right side.

Many persons with more serious sight losses such as those caused by cataract and glaucoma are afraid to attend a

motion picture, but others who have tried these simple rules
for correct viewing have enjoyed themselves and benefited
their sight.

TELEVISION

Much has been written and said about television's harmful
effects on sight. Many people who complain that television
is "straining" their eyes are trying to make every face, person
or object seem clearly etched. Actually, the images on the
screen are not sharply black and white. There is some blurring. It is not harmful to accept blurred vision. The harm
comes from straining to clear it.

Television has motion, and if you view it properly, it can
help improve your mobility and aid your vision in much the
same manner as motion pictures. Keep shifting the gaze.
Don't try to see the whole screen at once. Outline figures,
faces and objects.

Be certain to have a light on in the room. If the only
illuminated spot is the screen, your gaze will be riveted there.
If there is a lighted lamp in the room, your gaze will tend
to leave the television set fairly often to look at the light or
at objects in the room. This change of focus is part of good
seeing and restful for the eyes.

It's helpful to look away often to something in the distance.
If no distant view is available, hang a picture with a distant
perspective over the set and look at it frequently.

You'll find it helpful, too, to walk around the room or
into another room occasionally during an extended viewing.
Variety of seeing is important to sight.

If you are nearsighted, don't always look at the screen with
your glasses on. Try taking them off. Do your viewing
closer to the screen if necessary, but not closer than six
feet. Then as sight clears, move back even if it is only one
inch at a time. Eventually, you should be able to see the
program without glasses at the same distance as your

normally sighted friends. If you are farsighted, try watching the screen without glasses from clear across the room and gradually move closer to it, but not closer than 6 feet.

Finally, don't forget to rest your eyes with sunning and palming. A few minutes of each will give you the renewed vigor of sight necessary to view another program. Sun and palm, too, after you have finished a TV session. If possible, during the palming, do mental imagery that stresses distance and color, such as driving down a country road during the autumn season or taking a trip by boat along a beautiful coastline. You'll find this relaxing and restful.

View it properly, and television can help build your sight.

CONCERTS AND LECTURES

Concerts and lectures may put a strain on vision, but much of this can be avoided and sight built if a few suggestions are followed.

Watching a singer or a lecturer is the greatest hazard. There is little movement on the stage. You may find yourself staring—and straining to see the vocalist's or lecturer's facial expression. Look occasionally at the singer's accompanist. Watch the movement of his hands on the keyboard. Shift your gaze about the stage and let it rove over the audience. Change focus by looking down at your hand occasionally, or over to the person seated next to you. Close your eyes now and then.

If there's an intermission, leave your seat and walk around. Offer new stimuli, particularly various colors, to your eyes, and you will resume your seat with a renewed interest in the concert and with better sight potential.

Plays are much easier on the vision because they offer movement and color. Keep your gaze moving from actor to actor. Now and then, glance at something near at hand—perhaps the ear of the person in the seat ahead of you. Close your eyes occasionally, too.

If you will make use of these simple practices to insure relaxation, mobility and accommodation, you should enjoy a concert, lecture or play more, leave it with less fatigue, and you will be helping to build your vision.

MOTORING

Riding in a car, as driver or passenger, offers many opportunities for building sight.

An important caution: *Do not drive without your glasses until you have passed your state's driver's test without glasses.* It is illegal in some states to drive your car without your glasses if your license is marked "Restricted."

As you drive along, now and then shift your gaze from the road ahead to the oil gauge, then sweep your glance across the road again and then down at the speedometer. You'll notice less fatigue, and the change in focus should help to avoid a kind of hypnotic effect that constant staring at the highway ahead may have.

If there's a painted line down the middle of the road, shift your gaze from one side of it to the other. Follow it out, too, into the distance then shift to something close in the car.

At night, avoid looking directly at the headlights of oncoming cars. Instead, look at the right side of the road and then to one of the faintly illuminated dials on the dashboard. If headlights still bother you, try this simple aid: Before starting to drive, turn on your own headlights, stand about ten or fifteen feet in front of them with eyes closed and gently swing your head back and forth. Many persons have reported that after two minutes of this sunning they have been able to do an hour's night driving without being unduly bothered by oncoming lights.

If your distance sight is poor and you wish to improve it, sit beside the driver with your glasses off. Look out at the distant road and then at the oil gauge, and to the road again and then to the speedometer. Do a lot of counting. Count trees or houses or any other objects that come into view. As a passenger, you have more time than the driver to look around.

If you're farsighted you can use objects in the car as aids in increasing your close point vision—dials on the dashboard, for example. If you're a passenger instead of the driver, look off into the distance, then shift from one close object to another—the various dials, your fingers, etc.

Many people with a tendency to "car sickness" have reported that the suggestions for shifting given here have helped. If you are in motion—in plane, train, automobile, bus, subway or boat—staring fixedly at some object may often bring on motion sickness. Shifting may help avoid the discomfort. So may palming every now and then.

SPORTS

Viewing such sports as basketball, Ping-pong, baseball, tennis, jai alai and badminton can help build vision. The flight of ball or bird and movement of the players provide opportunity for fast visual shifting.

When you're at a baseball game, for example, watch the windup of the pitcher, the flight of the ball to the batter, the swing and hit, the fielder running toward the ball, the ball itself, the batter running to first base and the throw to first.

Participation in sports can be beneficial to vision. During the war when I helped prospective enlistees to bring sight up to service requirements, I advocated that they take an active part in sports such as tennis and basketball. If you're to play well, you must keep your sight moving—and that will help to build it.

GAMES

You can use card and other games to help improve your sight. With the exception of jigsaw puzzles, chess and checkers, which generally promote staring and are not advisable, most games provide opportunity for increasing mobility. Those which make use of dice are especially good for the purpose.

Try to play without your glasses. Do so for brief periods at first, gradually increasing the time. Keep your sight mobile; as you shuffle a deck of cards, watch the cards move. Dart your glance from one card to another as it is being dealt in a bridge game or as you lay out your solitaire game. Change focus often. Look from your cards to the face of another player; look around the room. Occasionally, do some vertical shifting—up and down a distant doorway or drape. Sometimes, when a new hand is being dealt, walk around the room briefly to relax your body and sight.

When you're playing with others and your eyes become tired, put your glasses back on for a while, take them off again later. When your vision tires and you're playing alone —in solitaire, for example—rest by sunning and palming for a few minutes, then go on with the game.

These simple rules will not interfere with your enjoyment of games and they'll make them valuable for speeding your sight improvement.

Introduction to the Step-by-Step Chapters

The techniques described in the preceding chapters provide the tools with which many types of vision deficiency can be —and have been—overcome.

Here, now, among the chapters in this section, you will find one which applies to your particular problem.

If you are nearsighted or farsighted, if you wear bifocals and have suffered a loss of vision both at the near and far points, if your problem is a crossed eye, or color-blindness, or if it's glaucoma, cataract or another of the more serious eye problems, or even blindness—exactly how do you apply the techniques?

How do you start? How do you proceed from day to day and week to week? Which techniques do you use—when— and what modifications, if any, will make them more valuable for your particular difficulty?

In one of the following chapters, you will find specific answers to your questions. Along with a brief discussion of your problem, there is a basic twelve-week program, which will show you exactly which techniques to use and the order in which to use them, daily, in each week. There are suggestions, also, for continuing the work beyond the twelve-week period, if necessary.

You'll find one or more case histories, too—examples of how others with your problem have progressed. They are included, first of all, because of their inspirational value. In addition, you may find that they offer further clarification of how vision can be improved.

In the absence of results from those who will read this book and employ these techniques on their own, I have had to use case histories of people who have been under my personal instruction. They worked at home, of course. In most cases, instruction was given once weekly, and all during the week practice of the techniques was done without supervision—as you will do them.

It is unquestionably easier to build your vision under the supervision of an experienced teacher. Progress is faster, too. The teacher can explain and demonstrate, make certain that the techniques are being used correctly and encourage and inspire. I would not be honest if I did not recommend that you find one of my qualified teachers.

However, in the earlier chapters and now in your step-by-step chapter, too, every effort has been made to explain clearly what you should do. While there is no substitute for a good teacher, you can use these techniques by yourself. You may not progress as rapidly as did some of the people I tell about, but you can expect to make good progress on your own.

All distances given in case histories are approximate as I do not measure.

Many of my students go to doctors more frequently than the average person, more than they would if they were not taking lessons, more than they would have gone before. I encourage these visits by giving them a free lesson each time a doctor decreases the strength of their glasses.

You will note that some of the people mentioned in case histories still wear glasses. If a person now sees as well with weaker glasses as he saw before his lessons with stronger glasses, I am pleased. If he now is able to see and work with glasses when before lessons he could not work either with or without glasses, his name is added to my list of successful cases.

Incidentally, you will find references in the case histories to extra equipment which you will not have to use. For example, in personal instruction, I use nineteen different letter boards of various sizes instead of the two which you may use. The largest letters are on my letter board No. 1; they're twice the size of your letter board No. 1. The smallest letters are on my letter board No. 19 and are one-fourth the size of your letter board No. 2. Your letter board No. 1 is equivalent to my letter board No. 9; your letter board No. 2, to my No. 15. I use the nineteen boards because they help, more graphically, to demonstrate improvement as the student progresses from one to the next. It is feasible for me to have this much equipment for use with many students. However, all nineteen letter boards—and other extra equipment I use—are not feasible for you. You have been told about the basic equipment you will need—and only what you will need. A minimum of equipment will save you time and money.

Some final general words of advice that apply to all vision difficulties.

Consider your lighting as you practice. You may need magnificent lighting at first, but if you are a nearsight or a farsight, gradually decrease the light until it is what is required by your normal-sighted friends. If light bothers you, gradually increase the intensity of light until you can take as much light as your normal-sighted friends enjoy.

If your improvement is not as much as you expected in any week, check your lighting to be sure it is not markedly less than it was the week before.

In any learning process, it is very important that the learner be praised if he does a good job. The small child walks better after his parents compliment him on his walking. The voice student sings better after being praised. If you work on your sight alone, compliment yourself. For example, after you have moved your letter board out another foot, or read smaller print and make this amount of gain, recognize that it is a gain, that you are progressing and that you deserve praise.

Remember how important the mind is in seeing. Above and beyond the mental factors we have already touched upon, there is an attitude of mind which deserves emphasis. The more you can actually think of yourself as seeing better, even as being a person with good sight, the more your sight will improve to match your mental attitude. You need a conviction in your mind that you are going to see better. Just as a man taking voice lessons visualizes himself, from time to time, as being on a stage before a vast audience and singing professionally, so must you see yourself as seeing well. You must see yourself as walking around with normal sight, working with normal sight and playing with normal sight.

Chapter XI

Step-by-Step
for Nearsightedness

Myopia, or nearsightedness, is perhaps the most common of all visual difficulties. About 60 per cent of the people who have taken lessons from me and my teachers have been nearsighted. They have ranged in age from six to eighty. The very great majority have benefited from visual re-education. Many who had worn glasses for twenty years or longer, requiring stronger and stronger lenses at frequent intervals, no longer use glasses at all.

If you are nearsighted, the techniques described in previous chapters will form the basis for your work in improving your vision. A few modifications, now to be presented, will make them even more helpful for you. And, with the step-by-step program outlined later in this chapter, you can begin immediately to improve your sight.

Your objective, as you know, is to stretch out your vision so that you will see as well at all distances as you do now at the close point. Let us re-emphasize this basic principle: It is not forcing which will do this, not straining and pushing. Relaxation is the key. It will unlock the door by relieving tensions that are a factor in your nearsightedness. In relaxed fashion, you will practice mobility and centralization, fusion and the other essential elements for good vision. Then, as you put them to co-ordinated use, your vision will move out to take in more and more distant areas.

RELAXATION

As a nearsight, you will benefit by doing the techniques of sunning and swinging just as described in Chapter III. No modifications of these are needed for your purposes.

An additional palming technique will be helpful. You will probably find that you gain a little extra relaxation, and afterward a little clearer sight, if you palm while lying flat on your back. Just why this seems to be of extra value to nearsights is not clear. Fortunately, however, palming in this position is easy and comfortable. You can do it before getting out of bed in the morning and just after retiring at night. A good substitute during the day is to palm as you lean back in a high-back chair. The back of your body as well as the back of your head should rest comfortably against the whole back of the chair.

You will note that the step-by-step program calls for you to spend a minimum of twenty minutes sunning and another twenty minutes palming each day. You can break up these sunning and palming sessions any way you like. It is often helpful to figure on four sessions of five minutes each. Certainly, you should do some sunning and palming the first thing in the morning and the last thing at night. It is a good idea, too, to sun and palm, even if only briefly, just before and just after doing accommodation drills.

When you practice mental imagery while palming, as described in Chapter III, you will gain most benefit if you visualize objects in color, working from near to far. Start by seeing in your mind an object close to you, then visualize others farther and farther away. Come back to the close one, then return to the others in the distance. Choose to visualize objects in motion as much as possible.

It will help if you practice mental imagery at times other than when you palm. Do some whenever you have the opportunity of closing your eyes for a few moments—during a pause in the day's work, on the way to or from work, during a TV commercial.

Two minutes of the long swing daily is a basic minimum. Do more, if you can. Remember to do at least a few long swings just before going to bed in order to make sure that you will not stare all night behind closed lids.

MOBILITY AND CENTRALIZATION

Just as in mental imagery practice, you will get best results from mobility and centralization practice by working outward, from near to far. When you count, for example, start with objects near at hand and move on to others as far in the distance as you can see. In outlining, start on large letters or objects near at hand—but go on to outline objects in the distance even if they're blurred. Do not worry about the blurring; outline as best you can. As you proceed with the other work, the blurring will vanish, but it is important to go ahead with the mobility and centralization drills with distant objects long before you are ready to see them clearly.

Many nearsighted people have a bad habit of rolling their eyes instead of moving their heads. Keep your head moving in all your mobility and centralization practice—and all day long as well. You must remember that a prime object of this practice is to build up your central and most sensitive vision. Only when you point your nose directly at what you want to see do you give yourself the opportunity to use central vision.

Many nearsighted people also habitually prop the head in one or both hands. If you do this, you lose mobility; you may also tense neck muscles and interfere with circulation. Try to break the habit as soon as you can.

FUSION

As a nearsight, you will benefit from working on fusion at all distances. Start at the close point—about a foot in front of the eyes—and work outward. Especially in the beginning, practice in front of a mirror in order to be certain that the cord, ring or other fusion device is being held directly in front of your nose rather than off at an angle. Fusion work at an angle is worse than useless. To train your eyes to converge properly, you must practice fusion directly out in front. Your head must be held level, too. If you tip it to one side so that one eye is lower than the other, fusion drills will be more difficult. A good check on "levelheadedness" is to see whether one of the two illusionary cords or doubled objects appears to be higher than the other. If it does, your head is tipped.

ACCOMMODATION

As you practice the accommodation drills, remember that these are designed to give you the opportunity to put into use all of the other techniques of good vision. You will see more clearly in the distance as you learn to see in relaxed fashion, with good fusion, and as your sight becomes mobile and centralized and you put the mind to proper use.

Sun and palm before starting your accommodation drills so you will be relaxed. Then work fast—with quick sight. For example, when practicing with the letter board, don't stare and try desperately hard. Use quick looks instead. Let the letters come to you. Don't be alarmed if the letters are blurred and you cannot tell the difference between *O* and *D*, *R* and *B*, *V* and *Y*, *C* and *G* and others somewhat similar in shape. This is where you use comparison and contrast. Be conscious of the white background. Slide along the white under the row of letters. If you are hunting *C* and come to a letter that might be *C* or might be *O*, close your eyes for a moment, think of white, then open your eyes for a fast look. Now the white background will stand out even more, and if you see white coming into the right side, you'll know the letter is a *C*. If you still have difficulty, look at an object beyond the board, then look back at the letter again.

You will need to use these methods each time you move the letter board farther away or practice other accommodation drills at greater distances. But when these methods have brought you to the point where you can, for example, see clearly all the letters at five feet, you will no longer have to make use of them at that distance, even though you will have to use them to stretch your sight to the six-foot mark.

All of this work is like learning how to do anything properly—even how to walk as a child. You must learn the proper basic habits, then learn to co-ordinate them, then achieve stability. You will have days in which your sight seems to be markedly improved; others in which it seems poorer. This is inevitable. Stability will come with further practice.

Some of your practice in accommodation will be devoted to reading. Many nearsighted people can read small print but have to hold it close.

In your reading, you will make use of ordinary reading matter—books, magazines, newspapers, etc.—plus the Gettysburg Address material in Chapter VIII (see p. 111).

Your effort will be to push your reading material farther away. You can do this in two ways. One method is to patch your stronger eye and read for several minutes with the weaker eye, with the reading material held in front of the patched eye. Then read for a lesser time with the stronger eye while the weaker one is patched, once again holding the material in front of the patched eye. Then read the same material for a few minutes with both eyes together. You will find now that you can hold it an inch farther away from you. As you continue this practice over a period of weeks, you will stretch your reading point out considerably.

In the second method, you use the graduated print Gettysburg Address material in Chapter VIII. Look first at Gettysburg Address IV. Hold it at a distance where you can see it without much difficulty and read the first two sentences.

Then read the same two sentences in V, the next smaller size print. Repeat with VI and VII—all held at the same distance. The smaller sizes may be mere blurs. But now turn back to IV again and it will be so clear that you can read it an inch to three inches farther away. Repeat the whole process, and next time around you will be able to move IV out another few inches.

MATTERS OF ATTITUDE

Do not be a perfectionist. Neither sight nor any of the other senses is perfect. Do not be alarmed if you make errors in calling letters. You are striving for improvement rather than perfection. Even the person with normal 20/20 vision occasionally misses a letter.

A person with normal vision uses his sight rapidly, without inhibition and does a good deal of guessing. He is unafraid and unself-conscious. For example, ask him to read at normal distance the capital letters *F-U-E-N-T-E* on a card, and he may call them *F - U - E - N - T - L*, then exclaim, "Oh no, that's not an *L*—it's an *E*."

Nearsighted people, on the other hand, often refuse to make a guess. Self-conscious, ever aware of their inability to see clearly, they stare hard rather than guess. The staring and loss of mobility may only add to the vision loss. Look briefly, say what you think you see, do not be afraid of an error, correct yourself when you see the need for a correction. But, above all, see without inhibiting yourself. In my teaching, I've observed that a salesman will usually regain his sight much more quickly than an engineer or a mathematics teacher. The latter are professionally trained not to guess.

STEP-BY-STEP

The step-by-step program covers a twelve-week period. In that length of time, you should make great progress in improving your vision.

Usually, at the end of twelve weeks, a nearsighted person who has been faithful in following the procedures outlined is ready for a change of glasses. If your sight loss has not been severe, if your vision is 20/40, according to your doctor, or approximately one-half normal, to begin with, you may, within the twelve weeks, attain 20/20 vision or close enough to it so you may need no glasses. If your vision loss is more severe, say 20/200 when you start, you will almost certainly need to continue for many weeks beyond this before bringing your vision up to normal or near normal. At the end of the twelfth week, it is usually a good idea to recheck your vision with your doctor and see if you should have another pair of glasses with a weaker correction.

When you've completed the twelve-week program, you can proceed with your own step-by-step schedule to achieve further improvement. As you will have noticed, each week's work contains balanced amounts of relaxation, mobility and centralization, fusion and accommodation drills. In planning additional practice, try to maintain the same balance. If there are certain techniques in each category which appeal to you and others which don't, make more use of those you like and less of the others.

By this time, too, if you have a weaker eye, you should have noted a difference in the rate of improvement in the one eye as against the other.

From now on, put more emphasis on improving the weaker eye.

BASIC TWELVE-WEEK PROGRAM
FOR THE NEARSIGHTED

Every day, every week:

1. Leave your glasses off when doing the drills. Go without them as much as you can at other times—but never

to the point of fatigue. Increase your "without glasses" time progressively from week to week.

2. Do the basic relaxation drills (see Chapter III)

    a. Sunning: 20 minutes in 4 sessions of 5 minutes each, or otherwise.

    b. Palming with visual imagery: 20 minutes.

    c. Long swing: 2 minutes.

    d. Short swings, one or two: 2 minutes total.

3. Count objects and colors (see Chapter IV) in free moments: as much as possible.

4. Edge objects (see Chapter IV) in free moments: as much as possible.

5. Practice vertical shifting (see Chapter IV) whenever possible.

Also each week:

1. See a movie and follow suggestions in Chapter x.

2. If you play cards, or other games, do so for increasing periods without glasses, and follow suggestions in Chapter x.

IN ADDITION
Practice each day during the

FIRST WEEK

1. Letter board No. 1 (Chap. vi): 5-10 minutes.

2. Cord fusion (Chap. v): 3 minutes.

SECOND WEEK

1. Domino wheel (Chap. vi): 2-4 minutes.

2. Alternate sunning and palming (Chap. III): 2 minutes.

3. Playing card drill (Chap. vi): one complete drill: 3-6 minutes.

4. Ruler shift (Chap. IV): 1-2 minutes.

5. Tossing ball (Chap. IV): 1-2 minutes.
6. Cord fusion (Chap. v): 3-5 minutes.

THIRD WEEK

1. Letter board No. 1. Patch and do a little more than half with weaker eye and the rest with the stronger eye (Chap. VI): 5-10 minutes.
2. Playing card drill, both eyes together (Chap. VI): 4-7 minutes.
3. Gettysburg Address (Chap. VIII) (see p. 111): 2-4 minutes.
4. Ring fusion (Chap. v): 2-3 minutes.

FOURTH WEEK

1. Solitaire, both eyes together (Chap. IV): 5 minutes or more.
2. Domino wheel, each eye separately (Chap. VI): 4-5 minutes total.
3. Letter board, both eyes together (Chap. VI): 5-10 minutes.
4. Watch to clock (Chap. VI): 1 minute.
5. Ruler shift (Chap. IV): 1-2 minutes.
6. Cord fusion (Chap. v): 3 minutes.
7. Ring fusion to letter board in distance (Chap. VI): 3 minutes.

FIFTH WEEK

1. Solitaire, with each eye separately and both together (Chap. IV): 5-10 minutes.
2. Letter board No. 2 (Chap. VI): 5-8 minutes.
3. Lights in mirror (Chap. IV): 3 minutes.
4. Ring fusion on jumbled numbers (Chap. VI): 3 minutes.
5. Perforated board sunning (Chap. III): 1-2 minutes.
6. Yardstick fusion (Chap. v): 2 minutes.

SIXTH WEEK

1. Reading, each eye separately and both together (Chap. xɪ): 3-5 minutes.
2. Letter board No. 1, each eye separately (Chap. vɪ): 5-10 minutes.
3. Jumbled numbers, both eyes together (Chap. vɪ): 2-4 minutes.
4. Cord fusion (Chap. v): 2-3 minutes.
5. Yardstick fusion to domino wheel (Chap. vɪ): 2-3 minutes.

SEVENTH WEEK

1. Lights in mirror (Chap. ɪv): 2-5 minutes.
2. Playing card drill, each eye separately (Chap. vɪ): 4-8 minutes.
3. Letter board No. 1, both eyes and together (Chap. vɪ): 4-8 minutes.
4. Near to far on magazine advertisements (Chap. vɪ): 2-3 minutes.
5. Ring fusion to letter board No. 1 (Chap. vɪ): 2-4 minutes.
6. Cord fusion (Chap. v): 3 minutes.

EIGHTH WEEK

1. Large red shifter in distance (Chap. ɪv): 1 minute.
2. Gettysburg Address (Chap. vɪɪɪ) (see p. 111): 2 minutes.
3. Jumbled numbers, each eye separately (Chap. vɪ): 5-10 minutes.
4. Letter board No. 2, both eyes together (Chap. vɪ): 5-10 minutes.
5. Plate fusion (Chap. v): 1-3 minutes.
6. Yardstick fusion to letter board No. 1 (Chap. vɪ): 2-3 minutes.

NINTH WEEK

1. Reading, each eye separately (Chap. xi): 2-5 minutes.
2. Reading, both eyes together (Chap. xi): 5 minutes.
3. Letter board No. 2, both eyes together (Chap. vi): 5-8 minutes.
4. Domino wheel (Chap. vi): 1-3 minutes.
5. Tossing ball and glancing out to red shifter in distance after each four tosses (Chap. iv): 2-3 minutes.
6. Plate fusion (Chap. v): 1-2 minutes.
7. Perforated board sunning (Chap. iii): 1-2 minutes.
8. Cord fusion (Chap. v): 2-5 minutes.

TENTH WEEK

1. Lights in mirror (Chap. iv): 2-5 minutes.
2. Gettysburg Address (Chap. viii, p. 111): 1-3 minutes.
3. Letter board No. 1, each eye separately (Chap. vi): 5-10 minutes.
4. Ring fusion to jumbled letters (Chap. vi): 2-3 minutes.
5. Toss cards (Chap. iv): 2-4 minutes.
6. Cord fusion (Chap. v): 2-4 minutes.

ELEVENTH WEEK

1. Letter board No. 2, each eye separately (Chap. vi): 5-10 minutes.
2. Playing card drill, both eyes together (Chap. vi): 3-6 minutes.
3. Jumbled letters (Chap. vi): 2-4 minutes.
4. Domino wheel (Chap. vi): 1-3 minutes.
5. Cord fusion (Chap. v): 3 minutes.
6. Card fusion (Chap. v): 2-4 minutes.

TWELFTH WEEK

1. Letter board No. 2, each eye separately (Chap. vi): 5-10 minutes.

2. Letter board No. 1, both eyes together (Chap. vi):
   4-8 minutes.
3. Large red shifter in distance (Chap. iv): 1 minute.
4. Ring fusion to jumbled letters (Chap. vi): 2-3 minutes.
5. Card fusion (Chap. v): 2-4 minutes.
6. Appointment with doctor.

Case Histories

Because nearsighted people vary so much in acuity of vision, three case studies are given instead of one.

David C. came to see if I could help him get into the Navy. His age was seventeen years and two months. At the Navy recruiting office, he had been able to read at a distance of only two feet a chart which should be read at twenty feet with normal sight. A doctor had confirmed the Navy finding of 20/200 or one-tenth of normal vision.

During the first two weeks, he took two lessons a week. In the first two lessons, the basic relaxation techniques of sunning, palming and the mobility techniques were taught. I also started him working, at four feet, the large letter boards, stressing speed. During the second lesson, too, I started using cards with rows of letters the size of those used by the Navy, about a half-inch high. At first I held them at two feet, moving back to three and a half feet. When he had trouble, I'd move up again and use a red pencil to point just over the tops of the letters, to keep his vision shifting. If the letters in a row were *A L C D L O Z T E* and he read *A L C* and then stopped, I would point rapidly at the letters and say "A L C 4 5 6 7 8 9" several times. This would clear another letter, perhaps the *E* at the end of the line. Then the pencil would make the shift from *C* to *E* while I said over and over, "*C* to *E*, *C* to *E*." The letters would begin to appear.

It was difficult to get him to guess what the letters might be. He wanted to see every one clearly before he called it. After two months when I finally convinced him that guessing was not "cheating," I moved back almost two feet in one lesson. As soon as he could see the letters at four feet, I gave him an eye patch and we worked the sight of each eye.

He was very co-operative about his homework. After the first two lessons he did not use his glasses for anything except to see the blackboard at school and to drive his father's car. Later, his teachers co-operated and he sat toward the front of the classroom to make it easier for him to read the blackboard without glasses. He stopped asking his father for the car except for an occasional date, and within three months he was almost never wearing glasses. The pair he had was now so strong for him that he said that he felt he had binoculars on the rare times he wore them.

He went to two, three or four movies a week, gradually moving back from the second row. When he had time he would see the same picture over, and during the second showing would move back five to eight more rows. His memory of it would help him to clear it.

During the winter, he turned out for basketball and played regularly without glasses. At home he played Ping-pong. When spring came, he turned out for baseball. He played the infield saying that in the outfield "it is tough to see."

He continued his home practice of fusion. He made use of anagrams for accommodation practice, and his mother helped by holding them and walking out farther from him. For this and for dominoes and mahjong drills, he wore his eye patch. In fact, he was so assiduous in patching that he wore out several patches.

During the two weeks before he was to take the Navy test again, he came to my office a half-hour a day just to read letters. He was reading letters now at distances varying from fourteen to eighteen feet. I knew, however, that he would not see that well under tension. A few days before his eighteenth birthday he passed the test at the recruiting office by reading the chart with each eye at ten feet. Thus he had

come from 20/200 to 20/40, or from one-tenth to half normal
vision. I heard from him several times during the period of
his enlistment. Each time he was retested, as at boot camp,
he wrote me a postcard telling me that he had passed again.
After the war he dropped in to tell me that he was still 20/40.

Mrs. M., another nearsight, was in her late forties and had
worn glasses for thirty-one years. Her vision had been tested
and diagnosed by her doctor as 20/200. Like David, she was
extremely co-operative. Immediately after her first lesson,
she began to eat meals without glasses and to do some of her
housework without them, too. Soon she was going without
them for all housework except, as she said, "I have to put
them on while I dust."

At home, she worked conscientiously with all the drills.
She had a view of a mountain in the distance. Often, she
would sit at a window, look at her thumbnail, then glance
out at the mountain. She made a game of trying to read signs
in the distance and license numbers of passing automobiles.
She was not too proud to wear an eye patch five minutes at
a time at the movies.

She played cards a great deal and, after the first two
months, played them entirely without glasses. One reason
for her improvement was the fact that she did not doubt it.
She never came to a lesson without commenting at once on
some improvement she had noted, such as seeing a clock
that she hadn't been able to see the month before. Eight and
a half months after her first lesson she passed the driver's
test with 20/40, or half normal vision. We then spaced her
lessons at once every two weeks until she read letters approximately a half-inch high from twenty feet with each eye.
Two years later, her driver's test was passed at 20/20. She
never wears glasses.

Mr. B. was an aviator worried about a recent loss of vision.
He'd been to a doctor and had been told that his sight had

dropped to 20/30. This meant, he told me, that the next time he took a vision test for flying he would be required to get glasses.

He was given the same first lessons, stressing relaxation and mobility techniques. Because of his relatively good sight, I started working letters at sixteen feet. At the end of the first lesson he was reading the half-inch letters at twenty feet. Also, because of his good sight, I did some near to far work with each eye and gave him a patch to take with him. He did a great deal of his practice standing because he said that he would have to stand during his test and that it was harder for him to see while standing than sitting.

The next week he reported that he had increased his distance on his playing card drill at home and felt he could see much better. At that lesson, seeing was speeded considerably so that there was little hesitancy on the half-inch-size letters. He tried reading at twenty feet letters approximately a quarter-inch high and did so with only one error with one eye and two with the other.

Two weeks later he had another lesson. Except for miscalling a few letters which he immediately corrected, he had no difficulty now in seeing with both eyes together all my quarter-inch letters at twenty feet. Then he read half-inch-high letters with each eye. With one eye, he read them at twenty-eight feet; with the other, at twenty-nine. Although I told him he didn't need any more lessons, he insisted on making another appointment for a month later. When he kept that appointment I stopped his lesson after half an hour; there was no need for more work. He phoned me a few weeks later and told me that he had read 20/15 with each eye for his flying test.

Chapter XII

Step-by-Step
for Farsightedness

If you see clearly in the distance but have difficulty in reading or other close point work—whether because of hypermetropia (plain farsightedness) or presbyopia (the farsightedness that's sometimes called middle-aged sight)—the program presented in this chapter is specifically for you. However, if you have also lost some acuity in your distance vision—if you have been wearing bifocals for some time—you may do best, instead, to follow the program in the next chapter which is designed to help improve both near and far vision.

Farsightedness is a common problem. It afflicts children as well as adults. More than three hundred of my students have been farsighted. Almost 90 per cent of them, young and old, have benefited from vision retraining, many to the point of being able to discard glasses entirely.

If you are farsighted, you will use all of the principles previously elaborated. You will improve your sight not by having to force it, not by straining to see things more clearly at the near point. Rather, you'll relax your eyes, your mind and your whole body, and rid yourself of habits of sight which, at best, do not aid it and may indeed be detracting from it. In relaxed fashion, you'll learn to make your sight mobile, to centralize it so you use the most sensitive area of the retina, to fuse it and to let your mind do its vital part of the job of seeing. And then, you'll put all of these proper habits into co-ordinated use to see more and more clearly at reading distance and even closer.

There are some modifications in the techniques previously discussed which will make them more helpful for you. There are a few special hints, too, which, as a farsight, you will probably find valuable. Then, with the step-by-step program that comes later in this chapter, you can begin immediately to improve your sight.

RELAXATION

No modifications are necessary in the techniques of sunning and swinging. Do them exactly as described in Chapter III. Just one caution: Many farsighted people with whom I've worked have tended to be volatile, quick in their motions, overactive and restless. If that's your temperament, watch for any tendency to move your head too fast from side to side while you're sunning and to swing your body too fast while you're doing the long swing. Make your motions slow, gentle and smooth.

When you palm, try often to visualize objects in motion, coming from far to near. Your ability to mentally visualize in the distance may be good even to begin with, because your distant vision is good. You may have a little trouble at first in visualizing things at the close point. The process will be easier if you first visualize something far away, then try to bring it in toward you, working ever and ever closer. For example, visualize a train approaching from the distance. You stand on the station platform and watch as it comes in. Or imagine you are walking toward a tree in the park and, as you draw closer, you see more and more fine detail until you pick a leaf off and, holding it in your hand, see the texture clearly.

Sun and palm as often as you can—any time you can, no matter how briefly. Practice mental imagery, too, as much as possible—even at moments when you may not be able to palm. Shut your eyes briefly on a bus or at your desk and visualize.

Some farsighted people with whom I have worked have complained of pain and discomfort, even with glasses on, when they read or sew for any length of time. As some have described the feeling, it's like "having sand in the eyes." If you have the problem, do the long swing even more than twice a day if you possibly can. Do the short swings—especially the lazy-daisy and cogwheel swings—more often, too. Do even more of the other relaxation techniques than called for in the step-by-step procedure. Your eyes will feel better and your sight will improve faster.

MOBILITY AND CENTRALIZATION

In your mobility and centralization work, the probability is that you will do better, at first, with distant objects than with close ones. You may have good mobility and centralization already when looking far away but tend to stare when you look at an object nearby, trying hard, in your anxiety, to see too big an area at one time.

All the techniques given in Chapter IV for mobility and centralization will be of value. You will find it especially important to practice them more intensively with objects near at hand rather than farther away. Do your counting at desk distance or even nearer, rather than clear across the room. For example, practice counting the capital letters in the title of this book, then the number of corners on each letter. Dump the contents of a box of matches on your desk and count them as you pick them up and replace them. Sweep across a line of print in this book and count the number of *t*'s, *e*'s and other letters.

Your edging, too, should be done most often at a normal reading distance, and you should work toward the point where you can edge small letters in a newspaper or book.

You may have to start with large headline type in a newspaper and work progressively toward the small body type.

A good practice is to take your glasses off when you use the telephone and doodle lower-case letters on a pad. Make an *a* on one side of the sheet, put a *b* on the other side and place other letters in random positions all over the sheet, moving your head as you do so.

FUSION

You will find it relatively easy to do fusion drills, too, at a distance, but increasingly difficult as you work them in closer to you. Yet all the emphasis should be on working from far to near. No matter how difficult near point fusion is for you at first, it will become progressively easier as you practice. And the quicker your close fusion improves, the quicker you'll obtain better close point vision.

Approach the fusion work in relaxed fashion. Stop when you're tired. Sun and palm for a few minutes, then try again. Don't expect perfection at once. If you get only brief flashes of what you should see, you're on your way. Gradually, there'll be more flashes and longer-lasting ones. Finally, after several weeks, you'll consistently be able to fuse well at the near point and print will be clear for you.

ACCOMMODATION

You will not need to use the letter board and playing card drills described in Chapter VI. These are more useful for increasing distance vision. You'll get best results with the other drills described in that chapter. In doing all of them— jumbled letters and numbers, clock and watch, etc.—work from far to near, looking out first into the distance then to the near point.

Keep your head moving, avoid staring, work quickly and easily. Don't expect perfection, don't attempt to force your sight. In this practice, you will be applying good habits of relaxation, mobility and centralization, fusion and mental sight. Be aware of them. Make sure you are using them. Your vision improvement will come as you learn in these accommodation drills to apply all these habits at once. Concentrate on the habits and let better sight come to you rather than straining to make it come.

Some of your practice will take the form of playing solitaire. This is a helpful method of improving mobility and centralization at the close point and good practice in accommodation as well. Many of my farsighted students have found it particularly valuable to use miniature cards. After using small cards for solitaire, they've found it much easier to go without their glasses while playing card games socially, using the regular-size cards.

Reading practice is an essential part of your program. All of it, as you know, is to be done without glasses. With each week's work, you will be moving forward, reading smaller print for longer periods, holding the reading material closer and closer to you.

Be patient with yourself. Start slowly. If, to begin with, you can practice no more than a minute or two at a sitting, fine. Try to get in the total time called for with a number of sessions each day. Later, you'll be able to lengthen the time of each practice session and cut down the number of them.

Review Chapter VIII. Remember to apply the aids given there to your practice reading.

It is important for you to eliminate any fear of not being able to see well. I have often been able to get farsighted people to a point where, during practice, they can consistently read print much smaller than that found in a telephone book. Yet these same people, handed a telephone book, are unable to read it. They freeze with fear. As you work with the techniques given in this book, your close point vision will progressively improve. You can help it improve much more quickly if you carry about with you a constant conviction not only that you are improving but that you will be able to read anything at the close point when you choose to.

STEP-BY-STEP

At the end of the twelve weeks of practice shown in the following program, the average farsight usually doubles his close point vision—that is, he can read without glasses print half the size he could read before. Many are ready at this point for a weaker pair of glasses. Some are able to do all their reading comfortably without glasses.

If you were one with a great loss of sight, you will need to continue practice. By this time, you will have seen which of these techniques seems to be most helpful to you. Concentrate on them now.

Just be certain, in drawing up any program for further work, that you include one or more drills in the four categories of relaxation, mobility and centralization, fusion and accommodation.

If one of your eyes has less acute vision than the other, put more emphasis on practice with that eye to bring it up to match the acuity of the other.

BASIC TWELVE-WEEK PROGRAM
FOR FARSIGHTERS

Every day, every week:

1. Leave your glasses off when doing the drills. Go without them as much as you can at other times—but never to the point of fatigue. Increase your "without glasses" time progressively from week to week.
2. Do the basic relaxation drills (see Chapter III)
   a. Sunning: 15-20 minutes in 4-6 sessions, or otherwise
   b. Palming with visual imagery: 15-20 minutes.

    c. Long swing: 2 minutes.
    d. Short swings, one or two: 2 minutes total.
3. Count objects and colors (see Chapter IV) in free moments: as much as possible.
4. Edge fine objects at the close point (Chapter IV) in free moments: as much as possible.
5. Practice vertical shifting (see Chapter IV): whenever possible.

Also each week:

1. See a movie and follow suggestions in Chapter X.
2. If you play cards, or other games, do so for increasing periods without glasses.

IN ADDITION
Practice each day during the

FIRST WEEK

1. Ruler shift (Chap. IV): 1-3 minutes.
2. Reading (Chap. VIII): 10-20 minutes total.
    a. Newspaper headlines.
    b. Magazine advertisements.
    c. Smallest Gettysburg Address possible (see p. 116).
3. Cord fusion (Chap. v): 2-4 minutes.

SECOND WEEK

1. Domino wheel (Chap. VI): 1-3 minutes.
2. Reading same material as first week: 15-20 minutes.
3. Jumbled letters (Chap. VI): 2-4 minutes.
4. Cord fusion (Chap. v): 2-4 minutes.

THIRD WEEK

1. Ring shift (Chap. IV): 1-3 minutes.
2. Reading (Chap. VIII)
    a. Each eye separately, smallest size print possible: 3-5 minutes.

    b. Both eyes together, including smallest Gettysburg Address possible (p. 116): 15-25 minutes.
3. Solitaire, both eyes together (Chap. IV): 5-10 minutes.
4. Ring fusion (Chap. V): 1-3 minutes.
5. Cord fusion (Chap. V): 2-3 minutes.

FOURTH WEEK

1. Ruler shift (Chap. IV): 1-3 minutes.
2. Jumbled letters, each eye separately (Chap. VI): 3-6 minutes.
3. Tossing dice, both eyes together (Chap. IV): 2-5 minutes.
4. Reading, both eyes together (Chap. VIII): 10-30 minutes.
5. Cord fusion (Chap. V): 1-3 minutes.
6. Ruler fusion (Chap. V): 1-2 minutes.

FIFTH WEEK

1. Domino wheel (Chap. VI): 1-3 minutes.
2. Reading (Chap. VIII)
    a. Each eye separately: 4-8 minutes.
    b. Both eyes together: 10-40 minutes.
3. Solitaire, both eyes together (Chap. IV): 5-10 minutes.
4. Jumbled numbers (Chap. VI): 1-3 minutes.
5. Cord fusion (Chap. V): 1-3 minutes.
6. Boat fusion (Chap. V): 1-2 minutes.

SIXTH WEEK

1. Small red shifter (Chap. IV): 1-2 minutes.
2. Reading (Chap. VIII)
    a. Each eye separately: 5-10 minutes.
    b. Both eyes together: 20-40 minutes.
    c. With red shifter under line of print: 1-3 minutes.
3. Jumbled numbers, both eyes together (Chap. VI): 1-3 minutes.

4. Cord fusion (Chap. v): 1-3 minutes.
5. Boat fusion (Chap. v): smaller boat than last week: 1-3 minutes.

SEVENTH WEEK

1. Ring shift (Chap. iv): 1-3 minutes.
2. Jumbled letters (Chap vi): 1-3 minutes.
3. Reading (Chap. viii)
   a. Both eyes together, with white file card underneath line of print: 1-3 minutes.
   b. With ruler fusion: 1-3 minutes.
   c. Other reading: 25-50 minutes.
4. Ring fusion (Chap. v): 1-3 minutes.
5. Plate fusion (Chap. v): 1-3 minutes.

EIGHTH WEEK

1. Perforated board sunning (Chap. iii): 1-2 minutes.
2. Domino wheel (Chap. vi): 1-3 minutes.
3. Reading (Chap. viii)
   a. Each eye separately, including smallest Gettysburg Address possible (p. 116): 4-8 minutes.
   b. Both eyes together, including page of graduated print: 20-50 minutes.
4. Plate fusion (Chap. v): 1-3 minutes.
5. Boat fusion (Chap. v): one large and then one small boat: 1-3 minutes.

NINTH WEEK

1. Alternate sunning and palming (Chap iii): 1-2 minutes.
2. Ruler shift (Chap. iv): 1-3 minutes.
3. Small red shifter (Chap. iv): 1-3 minutes.
4. Jumbled letters, each eye separately (Chap. vi): 2-4 minutes for each eye.
5. Reading (Chap viii): both eyes together: 25-60 minutes.

6. Ring fusion (Chap. v): 1-3 minutes.
7. Plate fusion (Chap. v): 1-3 minutes.

TENTH WEEK

1. Perforated board sunning (Chap. iii): 1-2 minutes.
2. Jumbled numbers (Chap. vi): 1-3 minutes.
3. Reading (Chap. viii)
   a. Each eye separately: 4-8 minutes.
   b. Both eyes together, starting with graduated print, then using book with large enough print so you can do speed reading: 20-60 minutes.
   c. With ruler fusion: 1-2 minutes.
4. Toss dice (Chap. iv): 2-4 minutes.
5. Plate fusion (Chap. iv): 1-3 minutes.
6. Cord fusion (Chap. iv): 1-3 minutes.

ELEVENTH WEEK

1. Alternate sunning and palming (Chap. iii): 1-2 minutes.
2. Domino wheel (Chap. vi): 1-3 minutes.
3. Jumbled letters (Chap. vi): 1-3 minutes.
4. Solitaire (Chap. iv): 5-10 minutes.
5. Reading (Chap. viii)
   a. Each eye separately, including graduated print: 4-8 minutes.
   b. Both eyes together: 20-80 minutes.
   c. With ruler fusion: 1 minute.
6. Boat fusion (Chap. v): 1-3 minutes.
7. Card fusion (Chap. v): 1-3 minutes.

TWELFTH WEEK

1. Perforated board sunning (Chap. iii): 1-2 minutes.
2. Ruler shifting (Chap. iv): 1-3 minutes.
3. Jumbled letters with one eye (Chap. vi): 2-5 minutes.

4. Jumbled numbers with other eye (Chap. vɪ): 2-5
   minutes.
5. Reading both eyes (Chap. vɪɪɪ): 30-80 minutes.
6. Ring fusion (Chap. v): 1-3 minutes.
7. Card fusion (Chap. v): 2-4 minutes.
8. Make appointment with doctor.

Case Histories

Mr. D., who had worn reading glasses for six years, was
a fifty-two-year-old accountant with a great deal of close
point work to do. He told me that without his glasses the
print was a complete blur. He came for lessons because, as
he said, "The glasses I have now are my fourth pair. Each
pair has been stronger and now I feel that I need another
stronger pair. Then, too, after my last examination I was
told that the next pair would be bifocals because of my age."

In his first lesson he was taught how to sun and palm.
The principles of mobility, curiosity, comparison, contrast,
memory and judgment were explained. He was shown how
to practice cord fusion and received a cord to take home
so that his wife or child could work with him. At twenty
feet the V of the cord was very clear, but there was only a
blur at eighteen inches.

The principles of accommodation were explained and he
was asked to practice the clock-to-watch drill.

In the first lesson, too, he was shown how to use and to
put emphasis on the white background, and was able to
read paragraph eight, on another graduated print set.

In his second lesson, the following week, the previous
lesson and his homework were reviewed briefly. Then he
was taught the ring shift and ring fusion and received a ring
to take home for practice.

Then I started him reading a book as fast as he could,
and at the end of each paragraph he would look up and read
a line or two of half-inch print across the room. Afterward,

he sunned again for two minutes. Then, on a different graduated print set, he read down to the smallest print. I helped to emphasize a margin-to-margin swing for him by tapping the white on one side of the line and then on the other with the tip of a red pencil.

In his third lesson, after a short period of sunning and palming, he was given an eye patch. With the left eye he read to paragraph eight and with the other eye to the smallest print in a graduated print set.

Then he did some reading at the distance for a rest, and some close point fusion. After this fusion with both eyes together he read all of the smallest type on a different graduated print set.

I asked him to work with the patch at home in reading practice and to play solitaire with each eye separately, then with both together.

When he came the next week he told me that his glasses were so strong that they hurt him. He said that he would go to his doctor during the week to see if he could get a weaker prescription. He phoned two days later that his new glasses would be one diopter weaker and that he was now doing part of his regular office work without glasses.

During his next lesson he was asked to read with the point of a red pencil sliding under the line. At the end of that lesson, he read the smallest graduated print with each eye separately and read several columns from a newspaper in a fairly weak light.

Two weeks later when he came for another lesson, he reported he was now reading newspapers entirely without glasses. During the lesson, he practiced on menus and telephone books. Half an hour was spent on close point fusion techniques. His next lesson was scheduled for a month later as he was going on a vacation. During his vacation he sent me a postcard on which he wrote: "Haven't had my glasses on!"

When he returned, he reported that his glasses were again too strong and that he had gotten a new pair, this time one-half diopter weaker than the previous pair.

His next lesson was his last. He had not had glasses on for two weeks and had no difficulty in seeing anything but the telephone book in poor light. He said, "It takes me a minute longer than most people to find a telephone number but eventually that will clear, too."

Not all people have the conviction of Mr. D. or apply themselves as conscientiously.

Mrs. H. J. had worn glasses for reading for six years and had recently had her second stronger pair prescribed. She had been told that the next change would be into bifocals.

Although she had two friends who had had lessons and discarded glasses entirely, she was extremely skeptical about her own ability to accomplish this.

She could read print comparable to Gettysburg Address II (p. 112), but at the end of the first lesson she was reading print comparable to Gettysburg Address IV. Yet, she kept saying, "I can't believe I'm really reading this."

For homework she was given a cord, domino wheel and jumbled number set. But a few days before her next appointment, she phoned to say that she "hadn't had any time to practice" and would come in two weeks later.

During her second lesson she explained that she was extremely nervous and didn't like to palm. When she said she liked music, I suggested that she palm while listening to music. At this lesson, she read print comparable in size to Gettysburg V after a great deal of relaxation work. The domino wheel and jumbled numbers drills were reviewed as she said she hadn't "looked at them." I gave her a set of jumbled letters and a ring for shifting.

The following week she complained that she had a head-ache so the lesson was not given.

At the next lesson she was able to get a few words of print comparable to Gettysburg VI but said working made her nervous.

The following week she saw print the size of the Gettysburg VI more easily, but as she was making so little progress I suggested she stop lessons, do some concentrated homework for a month and then return. She refused, saying she knew she could not do the work alone and needed someone to push her.

She kept on in this desultory fashion for some months.

She had great difficulty in getting ring, boat and plate fusion. It was difficult, although she liked music, to get her to move her head rhythmically.

At the end of eight months she was able to get a weaker pair of glasses, but has not practiced any further and still has to wear glasses for most of her reading.

Mrs. H. J. is not one of my star students. She did relatively little work and her progress was correspondingly small.

Mrs. E., a schoolteacher of about forty, had never worn glasses but had been given a prescription for reading glasses the week before she came to see me.

Her first lessons were exactly like Mr. D.'s except that she could read down to the smallest print when she came. She was given a cord and a ring to take home. She did much of her practice while attending to her school duties. She practiced accommodation with the clock in her classroom and her watch. She learned to shift rapidly over the ruled lines in her grade book to give her a faster shift at the close point. She used a ruler for the same purpose. She would hold it at her reading distance and then shift across the inch markings, then the half-inch lines and so on until the tiniest ones were clear.

She needed only three lessons and still reports that she has perfect sight although it is some years since she had lessons. She also reports that she still does a little fusion work occasionally and also suns and palms when her eyes feel tired.

Chapter XIII

Step-by-Step
for Bifocal Wearers

The program presented in this chapter is designed to help you if your problem is a loss of visual acuity at all distances which has made it necessary for you to wear bifocal, or even trifocal, lenses.

The great majority of people with this problem who have sought help from me and my teachers were farsighted first. They had been wearing reading glasses for some years, usually with several changes to stronger lenses before bifocals had been recommended. At that point, or soon afterward, lenses had been prescribed to help their distant as well as close point vision. There were a few who were nearsighted originally and subsequently suffered a loss of acuity in reading vision.

Almost 90 per cent of these people have benefited from vision retraining. More than one out of every three have been able to discard glasses entirely while the remainder need only weaker glasses for reading.

In your own case, your degree of improvement, of course, will depend upon the severity of your sight impairment when you begin and the conscientiousness with which you follow the program and the number of opportunities you seize all day long to practice better habits of sight.

You will make use of all of the principles presented in the earlier chapters. There will be no need to strain your eyes to see better. Instead, your improvement will come as you relax your eyes—and mind and even whole body—and, in relaxed fashion, learn to improve your mobility and centralization, perfect your fusion and make use of the other essential elements for good vision.

RELAXATION

You will benefit by practicing the techniques of sunning, palming and swinging exactly as described in Chapter III. No modifications are necessary.

In practicing mental imagery during palming—and it will be helpful if you practice this, too, at odd moments during the day when you can close your eyes briefly even without palming—you should visualize objects in motion, working out from close point to distance and then from distance in toward the close point. Thus, for example, if you're visualizing a train, picture it in your mind's eye as it moves away from you while you stand on a station platform. See it moving off into the distance until it vanishes from sight. Then picture it coming back—appearing far off on the horizon and coming closer and closer toward you until it arrives at the station.

If you're like many bifocal wearers, you may find that you tire fairly easily as you do the other drills called for in the program. Sun and palm for short periods in the midst of the drills, whenever you feel fatigue coming on, and you'll be able to continue, feeling refreshed.

MOBILITY AND CENTRALIZATION

Because your problem, like that of both the nearsighted and farsighted person, involves the need to build up central vision and mobility, you will use the drills described in Chapter IV. In counting, edging and all of the others—practice both at the far and near points. For example, you can count not only the petals in the flowers in a bouquet on your desk but also the flowers in the garden outside. Edge around a picture across the room as well as around a thumbnail. Balance your far and near work.

An additional mobility technique will be helpful if you have a special problem that bothers many bifocal wearers —droopy lids. To help overcome this, seat yourself comfortably in a chair, cross your legs and place the forefinger of one hand on the upper knee, holding it so it is straight in front of your nose. Hold the forefinger of the other hand about fifteen inches above the first finger and straight in front of your nose. Look at the top finger, then drop your head and look at the finger on your knee. Look up again at the first finger, with a head motion, and down again at the other. Do this four times with your eyes open, then four times with your eyes closed, remembering in your mind's eye the location of both fingers. Finally do the drill another four times with the eyes open again. You can profitably do this drill several times a day.

FUSION

The fusion techniques described in Chapter v will be of great value. Practice them at all distances. There may be certain distances at which fusion is particularly difficult for you. Start wherever you can in doing the cord fusion, for example, and work from there in both directions—closer to you and farther away. Do the same with the other fusion techniques. As you continue to practice, you can spend more and more time on the weaker areas of fusion until you improve at all distances.

Keep relaxed as you practice fusion. Look for gradual improvement, not immediate perfection. Rest often. At the slightest feeling of fatigue, stop and sun and palm briefly. The sunning and palming will send you back to further fusion practice rested and relaxed, and the relaxation will help bring further gains.

ACCOMMODATION

A few modifications in the accommodation drills described in Chapter VI will increase their value for you.

Before you begin to practice with the letter board, determine whether you can see, at a distance of ten feet, the smaller letters on letter board 2 on page 89. If you can, you need not bother to make up letter board 1 with the larger letters. Whenever a letter board drill is called for in the step-by-step program, you can work with letter board 2. If you must start with letter board 1, use it at increased distances and keep checking from time to time to see when your sight has improved enough so you can see letter board 2 at ten feet, then discard No. 1 and use No. 2.

In your letter board drills, because the letters you hold in your hand are large and you will see them more clearly than those in the distance, work from near to far. The same is true of the playing card drill. However, the jumbled number and jumbled letter drills will give you the opportunity to work both from near to far and from far to near, helping your sight at both distances.

The domino wheel drill also will provide good far to near practice. If you place the large wheel at a distance of three feet, and hold the small one in your hands out fourteen inches, you will probably find that the large distant wheel is clearer. Work from it to the small near wheel. If you're one of the few people for whom the distant wheel is more blurred, practice from near to far until the far one is clear, then you can reverse the procedure.

Much of your practice will be in reading. All the practice is done without glasses. Do it without strain and fatigue. If necessary, break up your practice sessions in the beginning so that you work even only a minute or two at a time. Later, you'll be able to lengthen the sessions, reading without your glasses with less and less effort.

If, like some bifocal wearers, you can read without difficulty with glasses off, print much smaller in size than that found in newspaper headlines or even magazine ads, there's no need to waste time with the larger print. Find print with which you do have difficulty—perhaps it's newspaper subhead type—and practice with that.

STEP-BY-STEP

The program which follows will carry you through twelve weeks of work. At the end of that time, it's likely that your vision will have improved enough so you will be ready to return to your doctor to be fitted with weaker bifocals or single-lens glasses.

And this need not be the end of the road.

If you were originally farsighted, once you can get back into reading glasses only, you will be ready to go on to do the work given in Chapter xii for the farsighted. You will be able to work toward the point, as many bifocal wearers have been able to do, where your vision improves enough so that you need to wear no glasses.

Similarly, if you were originally nearsighted, once you are back in single-lens glasses, you can do the work in Chapter xi for the nearsighted. Chances are good that it will help you enough so you will be able to discard the single-lens glasses or, at least, get weaker ones and, with still more work, eventually progress to the point of being able to discard your glasses.

BASIC TWELVE-WEEK PROGRAM FOR BIFOCAL WEARERS

Every day, every week:

1. Leave your glasses off when doing the drills. Go without them as much as you can at other times—but never

to the point of fatigue. Increase your "without glasses"
time progressively from week to week.
2. Do the basic relaxation drills (see Chapter III)
   a. Sunning: 4 sessions of 4 minutes each, or equivalent.
   b. Palming with visual imagery: 4 sessions of 4 minutes
      each, or equivalent.
   c. Long swing: 2 minutes.
   d. Short swings: one or more, 2 minutes total.
3. Count objects and colors (see Chapter IV) in free
   moments.
4. Edge objects (see Chapter IV) in free moments: as
   much as possible.
5. Practice vertical shifting (see Chapter IV): whenever
   possible.

Also, each week:
1. See a movie and follow suggestions in Chapter x.
2. If you play cards, or other games, do so for increasing
   periods without glasses.

IN ADDITION
Practice each day during the

FIRST WEEK
1. Letter board No. 1 or No. 2 whichever is possible at
   10 feet; if neither, use larger one closer to start (Chap.
   VI): 5-8 minutes.
2. Reading newspaper headlines and magazine advertisements or smaller print: 10-15 minutes.
3. Cord fusion (Chap. v): 2 sessions of 1-3 minutes each.

SECOND WEEK
1. Domino wheel (Chap. VI): 2-5 minutes.
2. Solitaire, both eyes (Chap. IV): 5 minutes or more.
3. Ruler shift (Chap. IV): 1-3 minutes.

4. Reading (Chap. viii): same as first week plus Gettysburg Address (see p. 111), if possible: 10-20 minutes.
5. Toss ball (Chap. iv): 2-4 minutes.
6. Ring shift (Chap. iv): 1-3 minutes.
7. Cord fusion (Chap. iv): 2 sessions of 1-3 minutes.

THIRD WEEK

1. If you can do letter board No. 1 (Chap. vi): at 10 feet, patch and do a little more than half with weaker eye and the rest with the stronger one: 10 minutes.
2. Letter board No. 2, both eyes together (Chap. vi): 6-8 minutes.
3. Jumbled letters (Chap. vi): 1-3 minutes.
4. Reading: (Chap. viii): 10-25 minutes.
   a. Gettysburg Address (a smaller size).
   b. "Seattle" card.
   c. Magazine advertisements.
5. Ring fusion (Chap. v): 1-3 minutes.
6. Cord fusion (Chap. v): 2-4 minutes.

FOURTH WEEK

1. Shifting on large domino wheel (Chap. vi): 1-2 minutes.
2. Jumbled numbers, near to far or far to near, working from the clearer to the less clear (Chap. vi): 2-5 minutes.
3. Solitaire (Chap. iv), each eye separately, then both together: 10 minutes or more.
4. Reading (Chap. viii): 15-30 minutes.
   a. Classified telephone directory advertisements.
   b. Book with large print.
5. Cord fusion (Chap. v): 2-3 minutes.
6. Plate fusion (Chap. v): 1-2 minutes.

FIFTH WEEK

1. Letter board No. 1 or No. 2 (Chap. vi): depending on distance you want to work: 5-8 minutes.
2. Reading (Chap. viii)
   a. Gettysburg Address (see p. 111) with each eye: 3-5 minutes, if possible.
   b. "Mental Sight" card with eyes together: 10-20 minutes.
3. Jumbled numbers (Chap. vi): 1-3 minutes.
4. Solitaire, both eyes together (Chap. iv): 5 minutes or more.
5. Ring fusion to board No. 1 in distance: 1-3 minutes.
6. Plate fusion (Chap. v): 1-2 minutes.

SIXTH WEEK

1. Domino wheel (Chap. vi): each eye: 3-5 minutes total.
2. Jumbled numbers (Chap. vi): both eyes together: 3-5 minutes.
3. Reading (Chap. viii): each eye, smallest print possible: 3-5 minutes; both eyes together: 15-30 minutes.
4. Ring fusion (Chap. v): 1-3 minutes.
5. Boat fusion (Chap. v): 1-2 minutes.

SEVENTH WEEK

1. Letter board No. 1 or No. 2 (Chap. vi): depending on distance you want to work each eye; 8-12 minutes total.
2. Jumbled letters (Chap. vi): both eyes together: 3-5 minutes.
3. Toss ball (Chap. iv): 2-4 minutes.
4. Reading (Chap. viii)
   a. Gettysburg Address (smallest size you can) (see p. 116) with each eye: 5-8 minutes total.
   b. Newspaper, with both eyes: 15-35 minutes.
5. Cord fusion (Chap. v): 2-5 minutes.

6. Plate fusion (Chap. v): 1-2 minutes.
7. Boat fusion (Chap. vm): 1-3 minutes.

EIGHTH WEEK

1. Jumbled numbers (Chap. vi): each eye separately: 3-5 minutes total.
2. Letter board No. 1 or No. 2, depending on distance you want to work, both eyes together: 5-8 minutes.
3. Domino wheel shifting (Chap. vi): 1-3 minutes.
4. Reading (Chap. vm): "Seattle" card or smallest print possible, with each eye separately and both together, followed by reading on white background: 20-40 minutes total.
5. Boat fusion (Chap. v): 1-3 minutes.
6. Cord fusion (Chap. v): 2-4 minutes.
7. Ring fusion to letter board (Chap. vi): 2-3 minutes.

NINTH WEEK

1. Letter board No. 1 or No. 2 (Chap. vi): each eye separately: 6-10 minutes.
2. Domino wheel (Chap. vi): both eyes together: 2-3 minutes.
3. Reading (Chap. vm)
   a. Each eye separately on Gettysburg Address (see p. 111) or smallest print possible: 5-8 minutes.
   b. Both eyes together on graduated print, plus newspaper or book speed reading: total 20-40 minutes.
4. Cord fusion (Chap. v): 2-3 minutes.
5. Small boat fusion (Chap. v): 1-2 minutes.

TENTH WEEK

1. Domino wheel (Chap. vi): each eye separately: 4-5 minutes each eye.
2. Jumbled letters (Chap. vi): both eyes together: 3-5 minutes.

3. Small domino wheel shifting, at reading distance (Chap. vi): 1-2 minutes.
4. Reading (Chap. viii)
   a. Newspaper: 20-40 minutes total.
   b. Book for fun.
5. Ruler fusion on graduated print (Chap. vi): 1-2 minutes.
6. Cord fusion (Chap. v): 2-5 minutes.

ELEVENTH WEEK

1. Letter board No. 1 or No. 2, depending on distance you want to work, each eye separately: 5-8 minutes.
2. Domino wheel (Chap. vi): both eyes together: 5-8 minutes.
3. Reading (Chap. viii): 20-50 minutes total.
   a. Telephone book.
   b. Telephone book with small red shifter.
4. Perforated board sunning (Chap. viii): 1-2 minutes.
5. Ring fusion on graduated print (Chap. vi): 1-3 minutes.
6. Ruler fusion on jumbled numbers (Chap. vi): 2-3 minutes.
7. Card fusion (Chap. v): 1-3 minutes.

TWELFTH WEEK

1. Jumbled letters (Chap. vi): each eye separately: 4-8 minutes total.
2. Jumbled numbers (Chap. vi): both eyes together: 2-5 minutes.
3. Perforated board sunning (Chap. iii): 1-2 minutes.
4. Reading (Chap. viii)
   a. Each eye separately on smallest Gettysburg Address possible (see p. 116).
   b. Graduated print and book or newspaper, both eyes together: 20-60 minutes total.
5. Ruler fusion (Chap. v): 1-2 minutes.

6. Card fusion (Chap. v): 2-3 minutes.
7. Make appointment with doctor.

CASE HISTORY

Mr. F., a sixty-five-year-old attorney, had worn glasses for sixteen years, beginning with reading glasses, then going to bifocals eight years before he came to me. He was concerned because he was getting a stronger pair of glasses every two years, and now, for the first time, he could not pass the driver's test without glasses. (He lived in a state whose laws provided for an eye test every two years in order to maintain a driver's license.) He reported that the inspector at the automobile testing station had told him that his distant sight was only 20/70. At the close point he could not read any of the graduated print sets without glasses, not even the top line or sentence.

In his first lesson, he was taught sunning, palming, the long swing, cord fusion, counting and the mental aspects of sight.

He did letter board 10 at approximately ten feet. For the close point, large cards with words half an inch high were used. He was told to try to play cards without his glasses. He felt very dependent on them but said he would play cards and eat meals without wearing them. He also promised to be diligent about his homework.

The following week he did board 12, a smaller board, and saw, at the close point, cards with words of smaller print than used during his first lesson. Because he could not do the ring fusion yet, we continued to use the cord fusion.

The following week he reported that when his wife was driving the car he would sit in the front seat with her, remove his glasses and imagine that he was driving. He also would try to extend his sight from one traffic light to the next and as far out as possible. He also reported that he was playing double Canfield with his wife and that the playing cards were becoming increasingly clear.

During his third lesson he read letters an inch high at approximately twenty feet but could not hold them clear. They would come and go, but he said that letters looked "less gray" than they had at the beginning.

When he arrived at my office a week later, he said he was not wearing his distance glasses except for driving and his bifocals only when in court. He also said that his eyes felt better and that he had noticed a decrease in his headaches. That was the first time I knew he had been suffering with headaches.

During that lesson he was able to do the ring fusion and was given a ring to take home. For the first time he was able to do the yardstick and ruler fusion successfully. For the first time he saw a few words on the top of one of the graduated print sets without his glasses.

A week later he was given an eye patch. With the left eye he did board 11 at about twelve feet, and with the right eye he did board 12 a little farther out. This was a big improvement over the first lesson when the best he could do was to see board 10 at approximately ten feet with both eyes together. He left, vowing that he would pass the driver's test without glasses in another six weeks.

The next four lessons were concerned mainly with work at the distance with each eye and with the two together. At the end of these four lessons, he did board 16 at almost twenty feet with both eyes together. In order to get these amazing results he had done the playing card drill with each eye every day at home. He said, "One night it was after midnight when my wife and I came home but I did my vision work anyway." By this time he was sunning and palming many times a day in his office as well as at home.

Two days later, he passed his driver's test without glasses. When he called to tell me this, I told him that we could now concentrate on close point sight.

The lessons, twenty-two in number, which he took to regain good reading vision would seem boring if told in detail. He worked down through weaker and weaker glasses until he could discard them entirely. We concentrated on finer and finer close point reading and speed of reading.

The last time I saw him he was reading novels, lawbooks, newspapers, menus and the telephone book, all without glasses.

Chapter XIV

Step-by-Step
for Crossed Eyes

If your eyes are crossed, in or out, the program offered here is designed to help you straighten them and to achieve better sight as well.

An experienced teacher is of great value particularly for the cross-eyed person. But if one is not available, you can proceed on your own with good hope of success, as long as you understand your problem and what you are trying to do.

Perhaps your eyes are not working together as they should so that they look in the same direction at the same time. The reason may be that the muscles which control the turning of the eyes are out of balance. Think of the problem not as being one of tugging and forcing short muscles to lengthen, but rather of relaxing cramped muscles. As they relax and uncramp, you can accustom them—gently and easily—to working together harmoniously.

While you are doing this, you will also be working to build up the vision of the weaker eye. For, as you know from earlier chapters, one of a person's eyes must almost inevitably be weaker if both cannot, at the same time, focus on an image. Clearest vision is in the central area of the retina, but when the eyes are crossed, the central area of only one eye at a time can be used since most crossed-eye people can look directly at an object with only one eye.

Building up the sight of your weaker eye will actually help in the process of straightening your eyes. For when there is a marked difference in the visual capacity of the eyes, there may be a strong tendency to keep using only one eye at a time for seeing—the stronger eye. The weak one may then turn out of focus.

Closely linked with straightening the eyes and building up the sight in both is the process of establishing fusion. As you learn, by fusion practice techniques, how to make the eyes converge properly in seeing an object, you will also learn to develop the power of the mind to properly fuse the two images sent to it from the eyes into one clear and perfect image.

This, in broad outline, is your program. The techniques you will use are, with some modifications, those you have read about in earlier chapters. They are not difficult to understand. But some of them, in your case, will be difficult to apply in the beginning. However, with patience you will be able to apply them.

Achieving straightened eyes and, with them, good vision is not a quick process. But the goal is worthwhile.

YOUR ANGLE

One of the very first steps is to determine your individual "angle" and put it to use, not only in your practice but at all other times. It has a cosmetic value, helping to make the eyes *look* straight to others. It also helps them to straighten.

You'll be able to learn your angle with the help of a friend. Suppose that, in your case, your left eye is turned in toward the nose. If you turn your *head* slightly to the right when you want to see an object directly ahead, you will then have to turn both *eyes* a little to the left to look at the object. At this angle, your eyes will appear to be straighter; they will have a parallelism that they don't have when you point your nose directly at what you want to see. Also, you will be coaxing the convergent left eye to turn outward.

You should use this angle in doing all your seeing and also, wherever applicable, in practicing the retraining techniques. As you progress, you will be able to shorten the angle, turning your head away less and less, until finally you will no longer need to turn away at all but can look, with both eyes in parallel, straight ahead at what you want to see.

To determine your proper angle, sit down, face to face, with a friend. Look directly at him, then very slowly, still looking at him as you do so, turn your head away. After a little experimenting, you will reach a point at which your eyes will appear to be straight. This is your particular angle. Have your friend tell you where your nose is now pointing —for example, toward the tip of your shoulder or perhaps halfway. With a little practice, while your friend checks, you should be able to establish this angle clearly in your mind.

If your right eye is turned in, your angle will, of course, be toward the left. It will be there, too, if the left eye is turned out. If the right eye is turned out, your angle will be to the right.

This is your beginning angle. As already indicated, as you make progress you can and should shorten the angle. In all likelihood, the time for this will come at the end of the twelve weeks' work given below. At this point, ask your friend to help again and recheck your angle.

RELAXATION

Your program calls for a considerable amount of time to be spent in practicing relaxation techniques. The sunning, palming and long swing should be done exactly as described in Chapter III.

In your mental imagery practice, when you palm remember to make use of your angle. By seeing things at an angle even with your eyes closed, you will be helping to straighten them.

You will find two special swing techniques of great value in helping to achieve relaxation and to straighten the eyes.

THE MIRROR SWING

Stand with your back to a mirror. If your left eye turns in, cover your right eye with one hand and look straight ahead

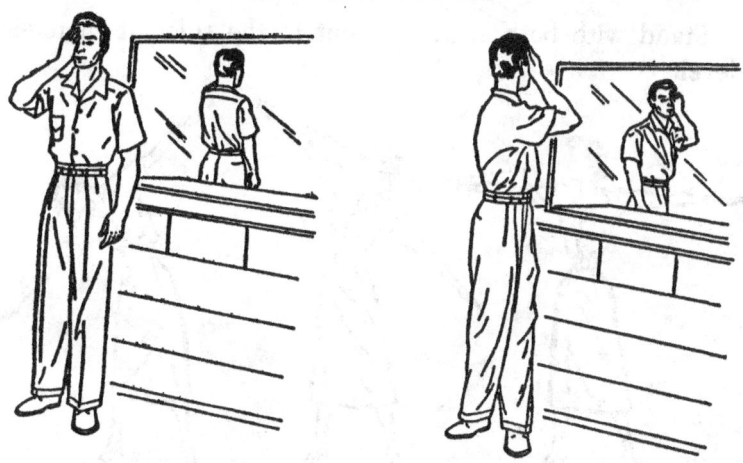

Fig. 35   Mirror Swing

with your left eye. Turn the upper half of your body to your left, letting your gaze drift with the movement of your body, until you see your left eye in the mirror, then return to the starting position. (See Fig. 35.) Do this four to six times. Next, cover your left eye and turn right to see the right eye in the mirror. Do this two or three times.

If your right eye turns in, do the drill four to six times with your left eye covered, turning right until you see the right eye in the mirror. Then do it two or three times with your right eye covered, turning left.

If your left eye turns out, cover your right eye and swing toward your right until you see the corner of your eye in the mirror. Do this four to six times and then cover your left eye and swing twice to your left, until you see the left eye in the mirror.

If your right eye turns out, cover the left eye and swing four to six times toward the left; then, with the right eye covered, swing twice to your right.

BALANCE SWING

Stand with both arms held out to the sides at shoulder level.

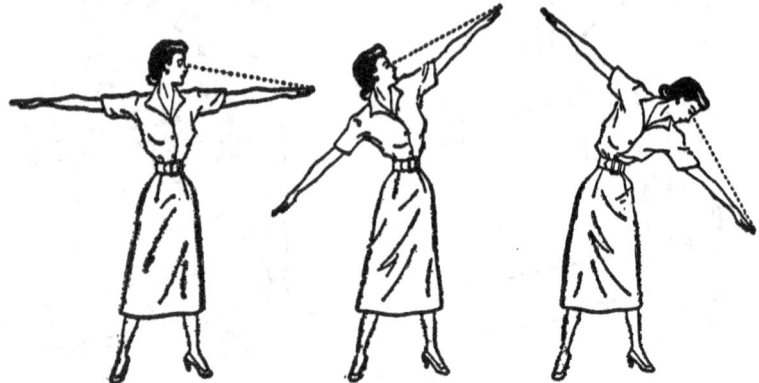

Fig. 36   Balance Swing

If your left eye turns in, or your right eye turns out, turn your head to the left. Bend the upper part of your body to the right, raising your left arm toward the ceiling and lowering the right arm toward the floor. Straighten, then bend to the left, lowering the left arm now and raising the right. Keep watching the left hand as your head and body move. (See Fig. 36.) Do this six or eight times. Then turn your head and do the drill twice while watching the right hand.

If your right eye turns in, or your left eye turns out, do the same drill, but turn your head to the right and watch the right hand six to eight times, then do it twice with head turned to the left, watching your left hand.

MOBILITY AND CENTRALIZATION

The techniques for mobility and centralization called for in the step-by-step program are done as described in Chapter IV, with just one modification. Do them at your angle. Instead of looking directly at objects you're counting or edging, turn your head slightly to one side so that you encourage straightening of the deviated eye. Do the same in the shifting drills with yardstick, ruler, etc.

If your case is complicated by the presence of nystagmus, uncontrolled oscillation of the eyes, omit the drills on the long red shifter, ruler, yardstick and ring and spend the time on extra sunning and fusion.

A special directional mobility drill with the large domino wheel will be of value. Wear an eye patch on your straight eye. If your left eye turns in or your right eye turns out, look with a head motion from the one-spot at the center of the wheel to the first domino at the left of the twelve o'clock position on the rim. Then, look back to the one in the hub. Now, look to the second domino to the left of the twelve o'clock position on the rim. Continue from hub to rim until you have covered the whole left side of the rim to the six o'clock position. The domino wheel should be held at a distance of twelve to eighteen inches in front of your eyes and there should be a head motion. Then put the patch on the deviating eye and repeat the drill, working to the right, from the twelve to the three o'clock position.

If your right eye turns in or your left eye turns out, work this drill on the right side of the rim, from the twelve o'clock to the six o'clock position. Then, with the other eye, work the left side from the twelve o'clock back to the nine o'clock position.

Another good technique which helps to straighten the

eyes and also increase mobility is to set up a string of five Christmas tree lights on a card table three feet in front of you. You will need a fairly sizable mirror. Perhaps it would be most practical to work in front of a door mirror. The mirror should be far enough away from the card table so you can get the reflection of five lights.

Look directly at the first light on the left, turning your head to the left. Then look in the mirror and find there the reflection of the third light. Then turn your head to the right and look directly at the fifth light. Then reverse, going back to look at the third light in the mirror and then directly at the first light. Continue to do this for two or three minutes.

Then look at the first light on the left in the mirror, directly at the third light in front of you, and finally at the fifth light in the mirror. Do this alternate method for two or three minutes.

FUSION

Achieving good fusion is one of the most difficult problems faced by the cross-eyed person. You will use techniques described in Chapter v.

Do not be alarmed if you are unable to do well all of those called for in the twelve weeks' program. Some cross-eyed people are able to achieve only cord fusion in that time. One woman who now has straight eyes took a year to get ring fusion although she could do all the others.

In beginning your cord fusion practice, tie one end of the cord to a doorknob and seat yourself three feet away. The tied end should be slightly below eye level (about six inches). Holding the tube at the other end of the cord with your right index finger and thumb, place it on the bridge of your nose exactly at eye level.

With your left hand, hold a file card over the left eye so you can see the cord only with the right eye. Now look at the far end of the cord and notice its position in relation to the objects alongside or beyond it. Notice how the cord cuts across the paneling in the door, or a design on the wallpaper to your left. Then transfer the file card to cover the right eye and look at the far end of the cord with your left eye. Notice that the cord now cuts across objects which are on your right-hand side instead of those on your left. Pay careful attention to the position of the cord in relation to these objects.

Next, close your eyes and form a clear mental picture of what you have just seen with the left eye. Focus, mentally, on the far end of the cord and all the objects it cuts across. (You may have to reopen your eyes several times for this, but do not be content until you have a very *clear mental* picture.) Keeping your eyes closed, move the file card to cover the left eye and now form a similar clear mental picture of what you have seen before with the right eye. Remove the card but keep your eyes closed a moment longer and mentally put together the two positions of the cord so that you see in your mind's eye two cords coming together to a point at the far end.

When you have a *clear* mental picture of how the "two" cords cut across the various objects in the visual field and come to a point, open your eyes and you should see—most likely only for a moment—what you have seen in your mind's eye. For that brief moment, you have had fusion; in that moment you have laid the foundation for better sight!

If the cord appears to be an X or a Y, you have still achieved some degree of fusion, but you may be focusing somewhere short of the end of the cord. Repeat the practice until you see the two cords forming the V. Do not be discouraged if you can only get a flash of the double cord and are unable to hold it for long. As you continue to practice, fusion will improve and hold for longer periods.

Once you have learned to work the cord fusion technique,

you can make use of it to help achieve more advanced fusion techniques. For example, if you have difficulty with ring fusion, tie the cord six feet away, look at the far end until you get the point of the V there, with the illusion of two cords coming up to your eyes. Then, slip the ring up alongside the cord. Continue looking at the end of the cord. If the cord is still double, you will now find that the ring is double, too, because it is right up against the cord.

If you cannot get the point of the V with a yardstick or ruler, you can employ the same technique. Once you've sighted along the cord and established the point of the V at the end of it with the two cords coming up to your eyes, simply slip your ruler or yardstick along the cord and, if you are still fusing on the cord, you will have to fuse on the other. You can do the same with the boat fusion technique.

If plate fusion is difficult for you, hold the plate either above or below the cord, with the center of the plate touching the cord. If you can see the point of the V of the cord through the two holes, then you will get an optical illusion of three holes.

One additional fusion technique is included here because it is of particular value for crossed eyes.

While seated, hold a yardstick with the one end just below your nose and the other end pointed straight away from you. Get a V on this as described in Chapter v. Now, keeping the V, swing your head and the yardstick to right, and to left, then up and down.

ACCOMMODATION

All of the techniques given in Chapter vi will be of value in improving your visual acuity at all distances and in helping to equalize the sight in both eyes. Do not be disturbed if middle letters of words close to you or middle letters on the letter board in the distance blank out sometimes. Almost all people with crossed-eye problems experience this at first. As your sight improves, however, you will find that there is less and less blanking out.

MENTAL AIDS

Follow the techniques described in Chapter vii. All will be of value. Memory of perfect sight will help bring more perfect sight. And memory of straight eyes will help to straighten your eyes.

Have a friend or relative tell you when your eyes look straight. Note how they feel at that time. Later, whenever you know your eyes are crossing, close your eyes and remember how they felt when they were straight. When you open them again, they should look straight again. This, incidentally, is an excellent technique to use just before you have a picture taken.

STEP-BY-STEP

The twelve-week program that follows will start you along the road toward straightening your eyes, achieving good fusion and improving your vision in both eyes at all distances. It is not an easy or short road. At the end of the twelve weeks, you may have progressed to where, for hours and possibly even days, your eyes will be perfectly straight. However, achieving permanent straightness usually requires further work. It is not at all unusual for a person with severe crossing to have to work for a year and even eighteen months before he can establish all of the good seeing habits so firmly that there will be no tendency to revert to crossing again.

When you have completed the twelve weeks' work, you should have achieved sufficient straightening of the eye so that you can shorten your angle. Use the new angle in further practice.

You can continue practice using the twelve weeks' work as a basis or you can make some changes. You should devote

the same over-all time to each of the categories of work—
that is, relaxation, mobility and centralization, fusion, accommodation. In all except fusion, you can vary the work, using
those particular techniques in each category which happen
to be your favorites and which you find most helpful.

In fusion, however, all of the emphasis must be on using
the more advanced techniques. If at the end of twelve weeks,
you are still able to do well only the elementary fusion techniques, you should continue on to practice the more advanced
techniques until you can use them with the same proficiency
you've achieved in cord fusion.

This will help you to continue should you become discouraged with slowness of fusion. I have many photographs
(before and after) of people who were crossed but now
look at the world and their friends with straight eyes.

BASIC TWELVE-WEEK PROGRAM
FOR CROSS-EYES

Every day, every week:
1. Do the basic relaxation drills (see Chapter III)
   a. Sunning: 20 minutes in 4 sessions of 5 minutes each.
   b. Palming with visual imagery: 6 sessions, 4 minutes
      each.
   c. Long swing: 2 minutes.
   d. Short swings, one or two: 2 minutes total.
2. Maintain your "angle" at all times possible.
3. Count objects and colors (Chap. IV) with and without
   a patch, using your angle: as much as possible.
4. Edge objects (Chap. IV) in free moments: as much as
   possible.
5. Toss ball (Chap. IV): 1-3 minutes.

Also each week:
1. See a movie and use your angle.
2. Play cards and other games, holding your angle.

IN ADDITION
Practice each day during

FIRST WEEK

1. Letter board No. 1 at angle (Chap. vi): all but 8 or 10 letters with crossed eye. Last letters with board for straight eye: 8-12 minutes.
2. a. Reading with crossed eye (Chap. viii): newspaper headlines or magazine advertisements, holding your angle: 3-5 minutes.
   b. Reading with straight eye (Chap. viii): book or newspaper: 2 minutes.
3. Red shifter (Chap. iv): 1-2 minutes.
4. Cord fusion (Chap. v): 1-2 minutes.

SECOND WEEK

1. Letter board No. 1 (Chap. vi): at angle, all but 8 or 10 letters with crossed eye, farther out if possible. Last letters with board in front for straight eye: 6-10 minutes.
2. a. Domino wheel (Chap xiv): directionally, ½ of one side with crossed eye: 2 minutes.
   b. Near to far on domino wheel (Chap. vi): with straight eye: 1 minute.
3. Reading (Chap. viii).
   a. With crossed eye, newspaper headlines or magazine advertisements: 4-6 minutes.
   b. With straight eye, book or newspaper: 2 minutes.
   c. With both eyes: 3 minutes.
4. Ring shift (Chap. iv): 1-2 minutes.
5. Mirror swing (Chap. xiv): 1-3 minutes total time. It should be done 5 times a day.
6. Cord fusion (Chap. v): 1-2 minutes.

THIRD WEEK

1. Playing card drill (Chap. vi): 5-12 minutes.

a. 40 cards minimum at angle, crossed eye.
b. Straight eye with board straight ahead, 12 cards.
2. Mirror swing (Chap. xii): 1-3 minutes.
3. Reading (Chap. viii)
    a. Crossed eye, newspaper headlines or magazine advertisements: 8 minutes.
    b. Straight eye, book or newspaper: 2 minutes.
    c. Both eyes: 5 minutes.
4. Ring shift (Chap. iv): 1-3 minutes.
5. Red shifter (Chap. iv): 1-2 minutes.
6. Cord fusion (Chap. v): 1-3 minutes.

FOURTH WEEK

1. Letter board No. 2 at angle (Chap. vi): all but 8 or 10 letters with crossed eye. Last letters with board in front for straight eye: 6-10 minutes.
2. Domino wheel (Chap. xiv): directionally, ½ of one side with crossed eye: 2-3 minutes. Near to far on domino wheels (Chap. vi) with straight eye: 1 minute.
3. Balance swing (Chap. xiv): 4 times with crossed eye; 2 times with straight eye: 1 minute.
4. Ring shift (Chap. iv): 1-2 minutes.
5. Reading (Chap. viii)
    a. With crossed eye: 5-8 minutes.
    b. With straight eye: 1 minute.
    c. With both eyes: 5 minutes.
6. Cord fusion (Chap. v): 1-3 minutes.

FIFTH WEEK

1. Jumbled letters (Chap. vi): 3-6 minutes.
    a. ¾ with crossed eye.
    b. ¼ with straight eye.
2. Balance swing (Chap xiv): 4 times a day: 1-3 minutes total.
3. Mirror swing (Chap. xiv): 8 times a day: 3-5 minutes total.

4. Reading (Chap. vIII)
   a. With crossed eye, newspaper headlines or magazine advertisements: 8 minutes.
   b. With straight eye, book or newspaper: 2 minutes.
   c. With both eyes: 5 minutes.
5. Solitaire (Chap. IV): 10-15 minutes total.
   a. With crossed eye, 1 game.
   b. With straight eye, ½ game.
   c. Finish with both eyes.
6. Ruler shift (Chap. IV): 1-2 minutes.
7. Cord fusion (Chap. V): 1-3 minutes.

SIXTH WEEK

1. Letter board No. 1 (Chap. VI): at angle—all but 8 or 10 letters with crossed eye. Last letters with board in front for straight eye: 6-12 minutes total.
2. Toss dice (Chap. IV): 2 minutes with crossed eye, 1 minute with straight eye.
3. Ring shift (Chap. IV): both eyes: 1-3 minutes.
4. Domino wheel, directionally (Chap. XIV)
   a. ½ of one side with crossed eye: 2 minutes.
   b. Near to far on domino wheels (Chap. VI): with straight eye: 1-2 minutes.
5. Mirror swing (Chap. XIV): 8 times a day: 3-5 minutes total time.
6. Balance swing (Chap. XIV): 4 times a day: 1-2 minutes.
7. Cord fusion (Chap. V): 2-3 minutes.
8. Plate fusion (Chap. V), using cord fusion as guide (Chap. XIV): 1-2 minutes.
9. Playing card drill (Chap. VI): both eyes together, holding angle: 5 minutes.

SEVENTH WEEK

1. Letter board No. 2 (Chap. VI): at angle, all but 8 or 10 letters with crossed eye. Last letters with board in front for straight eye: 6-12 minutes.

2. Jumbled letters (Chap. vi): ¼ with crossed eye; ¼ with straight eye: 6-10 minutes.
3. Reading (Chap. viii)
    a. With crossed eye, newspaper headlines or magazine advertisements: 8 minutes.
    b. With straight eye, book or newspaper: 5 minutes.
    c. With both eyes: 5 minutes.
4. Mirror swing (Chap. xiv): 8-10 times a day: 3-6 minutes total time.
5. Balance swing (Chap. xiv): 5 times a day: 1-3 minutes total.
6. Red shifter: 1-2 minutes.
7. Domino wheel, directionally (Chap. xiv): 1-5 minutes.
8. Cord fusion (Chap. v): 2-4 minutes. (Try ring fusion but do not be discouraged if you do not get it.)

EIGHTH WEEK

1. Letter board No. 2 (Chap. vi): 30 letters with crossed eye; 8 with straight eye; and 10 with both eyes: 15-20 minutes.
2. Lights in mirror (Chap. xiv): 2-4 minutes.
3. Mirror swing (Chap. xiv): 8-10 times a day: 3-6 minutes total.
4. Balance swing (Chap. xiv): 5 times a day: 1-3 minutes total.
5. Cord fusion (Chap. v): 2-3 minutes.
6. Red shifter (Chap. iv): 1-2 minutes.
7. Jumbled numbers (Chap. vi): with both eyes, but holding angle: 3-6 minutes.
8. Plate fusion (Chap. v): 1-3 minutes.

NINTH WEEK

1. Letter board No. 2 (at angle—all but 8 or 10 letters with crossed eye. Last letters with board in front for straight eye): 6-12 minutes.

2. Solitaire (Chap. IV): 3 games with crossed eye; 1 with straight eye; and 1 with both eyes together: 10-20 minutes.
3. Ruler shift (Chap. IV): 1-3 minutes.
4. Ring shift (Chap. IV): 1-3 minutes.
5. Mirror swing (Chap. XIV): 8-10 times a day: 3-6 minutes total time.
6. Balance swing (Chap. XIV): 1-3 minutes.
7. Cord fusion (Chap. V): 2-3 minutes.
8. Plate fusion (Chap. V): 1-2 minutes.
9. Try ring fusion (Chap. V): 1-2 minutes.

TENTH WEEK

1. Letter board No. 2 (at angle—all but 8 or 10 letters with crossed eye. Last letters with board in front for straight eye): 6-12 minutes.
2. Lights in mirror (Chap. XIV): 3-6 minutes.
3. Mirror swing (Chap. XIV): 8-10 times a day: 3-6 minutes total.
4. Balance swing (Chap. XIV): 8 times with crossed eye; 2 times with straight eye: 1 minute.
5. Reading (Chap. VIII): Gettysburg Address (see p. 111) with crossed eye the size that you can do: 4-7 minutes.
6. Book print reading (Chap. VIII); with straight eye: 2 minutes.
7. Ruler shift (Chap. IV): 1-2 minutes.
8. Solitaire (Chap. IV): 2 games with crossed eye; 1 game with straight eye; 1 game both eyes together: 8-15 minutes.
9. Red shifter (Chap. IV): 1-2 minutes.
10. Cord fusion (Chap. V): 2-4 minutes.
11. Ring fusion, laying ring alongside of cord (Chap. V): 1-3 minutes.

ELEVENTH WEEK

1. Jumbled letters (Chap. vi): ⅛ with crossed eye; ¼ with straight eye: 6-10 minutes.
2. Domino wheel, directionally (Chap. xiv): 4-6 minutes.
3. Toss dice (Chap. iv): crossed eye 5 minutes; straight eye 2 minutes.
4. Jumbled numbers (Chap. vi): ⅛ with crossed eye; ¼ with straight eye: 5-8 minutes.
5. Playing card drill (Chap. vi): at angle with crossed eye, 40 cards. Straight eye with board straight ahead, 12 cards: 4-10 minutes.
6. Reading (Chap. viii)
   a. Smaller print with crossed eye: 5 minutes; with straight eye: 2 minutes.
   b. With plate fusion or ruler: 1 minute.
7. Balance swing (Chap. xiv): 4 times a day: 1-3 minutes.
8. Yardstick fusion (Chap. v): 1-2 minutes.
9. Boat fusion (Chap. v): 1-2 minutes.
10. Cord fusion: 1-2 minutes.

TWELFTH WEEK

1. Letter board No. 2 (Chap. vi): at angle—all but 8 or 10 letters with crossed eye. Last letters with board in front for straight eye: 5-10 minutes.
2. Lights in mirror (Chap. xiv): 2-5 minutes.
3. Solitaire (Chap. iv): crossed eye, 1 game; straight eye, ½ game; both eyes, ¼ game: 5-8 minutes.
4. Domino wheel, directionally (Chap. xiv): ⅛ of one side with crossed eye: 2 minutes. Near to far on domino wheel (Chap. vi) with straight eye.
5. Reading (Chap. viii)
   a. With crossed eye Gettysburg Address (see p. 116) or as small print as you can: 5 minutes.
   b. With straight eye: 2 minutes.

6. Mirror swing (Chap. xiv): 5-10 times a day: 3-6 minutes total time.
7. Balance swing (Chap. xiv): 4 times a day: 1-3 minutes.
8. Cord fusion (Chap. v): 2-8 minutes (2 sessions).
9. Plate fusion (Chap. v): 1-2 minutes.
10. Yardstick fusion (Chap. v): 1 minute.
11. Boat fusion (Chap. v): 1-2 minutes.
12. Cord fusion (Chap. v): 1-4 minutes.

CASE HISTORIES

The case studies in this section help to give you a great many pointers. Three cases have been chosen, one convergent (eye turning in), one divergent (eye turning out) and one alternate crossing.

Mr. P., twenty-two years of age, was a graduate student at a nearby university. He said that his doctor's diagnosis was strabismus in the left eye with visual acuity of 4/200. The eye turned in. The right eye had 20/20 vision. He had worn glasses but had discarded them. The left eye had been operated on unsuccessfully twice, once when he was ten and again when he was fourteen. At sixteen, he had had a series of orthoptic treatments which he said had been unsuccessful.

In his first lesson, he was shown how to do all the relaxation techniques and taught his correct angle. His eye looked straighter after the sunning and palming. His right eye was patched, and with the left eye he did half of board 1. The right eye, the one under the patch, became tired so he was given another short sunning. With the left eye patched, he read small words from clear across the room, a distance of about twenty-four feet.

When the fusion cord was tried, he could get faint glimpses of the V off slightly to his right at a few inches, with the help of a light on his left side.

The following week, he reported that he had been holding his correct angle as much as possible and that he had been playing solitaire, one game with the left eye, and one game with the right eye, but that he had not had time to make up the playing card drill. With the left eye, he did board 1 a little farther out. His chair was placed at a slight angle to the right so that the left eye had a more straight look as he worked. After a short rest, the left eye was patched, and with the right eye he read small words from across the room. Fusion on the cord now extended out about twenty inches.

In his third lesson, a week later, there was further improvement in letter board 3 at about three feet, and this time he did all the forty-eight letters without either eye becoming tired. Cord fusion was extended out to six feet by means of mental imagery. (He would close his eyes and imagine how the cord should look farther out, then open and try to see it.) After a short period of sunning and palming and the mirror swing, he was able to hold the V of the cord for a longer period.

He reported that he noticed that his eye seemed better after doing the long swing. Now the balance swing was added.

In his fourth lesson, and then in all subsequent lessons, he did smaller and smaller boards.

Fusion on the cord was extended out to fifteen feet by the tenth lesson. We then went on to ring fusion. He also began to get the A, V and X on a ruler and later the channel.

Often when he would read with both eyes together, he would hold the point of a red pencil under the word he was focusing on. The end of the pencil toward him would double slightly and the pointed end seemed to be the point of a V.

After his twelfth lesson, he began to report occasional double vision. The eye which formerly hadn't worked was now coming into increasing use although fusion wasn't perfect enough yet. When doubling occurred, he would close his eyes and imagine he saw a single object. When this did not work, he would practice fusion. By the sixteenth lesson, there was no more doubling, and fusion improved. He was helped considerably in his progress because his family and friends kept noting his improvement. After his twenty-ninth lesson, a new acquaintance refused to believe that he had ever been crossed. When last heard from, he reported straight eyes and a visual acuity of 20/40 in the left eye and 20/10 in the right eye. He was playing tennis which he had never been able to do before. He was delighted by his social poise now.

Mrs. R., thirty-five years old when she came for her interview, had had a turned-in right eye as a child. Surgery had been performed at twelve. At twenty-two, the right eye began to turn out. When she would cover her left eye, the right eye would be straighter. She said that she had very little sight in the right eye, but that the left eye was 20/40 according to her doctor.

She came from some distance so she took a lesson every day for four days.

Her first lesson was the same as Mr. P's. There was more difficulty in finding her angle. She finally discovered that her nose should point slightly to the right and her eyes slightly left. She was asked to hold this position when watching movies, attending concerts and lectures and when conversing with friends. Only two glimpses of the cord and those slightly to her right were obtained on the first lesson.

Her sight in the right eye was too poor for even letter board 1 so large letters were used. She would hold them to her right and watch them as she moved them in front of her nose. The left eye was worked on the letter boards. At the end of her fourth lesson, she was fusing with the cord out to two and a half feet, but could not hold fusion for more than a few seconds. She was given a ring to take home for practice in shifting and taught the mirror swing.

When she came again a month later, she had a notebook to show how much she'd practiced. She had sunned, palmed and done the long swing and the mirror swing many times a day. Her husband had helped her with the fusion cord every day. She had tried to play solitaire, but the right eye could not see the cards that far away. So she'd gone through the pack of cards several times a day, calling them as she moved them from right to left in front of the right eye. She had made a playing card board and had done that drill at least once a day with the left eye.

Her vision seemed much improved and she did letter board 1 with the right eye at about two feet and board No. 12 at about fourteen feet with the left eye. She was able to extend her cord fusion farther out.

A month later she returned for two more lessons. She said that she had made a playing card board of miniature cards and was using that for the left eye, and the regular-size cards for the right eye. Her husband continued to help her with the fusion cord.

Two months later, she returned for two more lessons. This time she got touches of fusion on the ring. She said she had had some double vision, but she had remembered my suggestion to close her eyes and visualize single objects and to do fusion when doubling occurred. She also reported that her friends were beginning to comment on her improved appearance and she was enjoying her social activities more.

Two months later, she reported that her eyes were holding straight for periods of as long as half an hour at a time. She began to get the advanced fusion and said it made her "feel good."

She had four more lessons over a period of four months. At the end of that time, she took a driver's test, and was rated 20/20 in the left eye and 20/100 in the right. Her eyes kept holding straight now except when she was tired and upset and then she did a little fusion work.

John S., a man about twenty-five, had an alternate divergent crossing. He said there had been no operations and orthoptics had been unsuccessful. He said he had normal sight in each eye, although the right eye was slightly better than normal. The left eye turned in more often than the right eye when used for distance; the right eye turned in more often when reading.

He was given the same first lesson as the others, except that he was not taught an angle of vision because he could not always tell which eye was deviating. Cord fusion was difficult for him and he saw only two brief flashes of the V, until the cord was moved from side to side with his nose following it.

(His homework consisted of sunning, palming, long, short and mirror swings and playing card drill, working each eye at a slightly outward angle.)

On his fourth lesson, he was given ring fusion. After this, he began to play handball, then took up tennis, and badminton as well. He also patched and read with each eye separately and then with the two together. When he read with one eye alone, he would hold the book a few inches to the side of the eye in use instead of directly in front of him. In subsequent lessons, we progressed to the more advanced fusion. He needed only fifteen lessons over a period of a year to achieve what he felt was perfect fusion.

Chapter XV

Step-by-Step
for Color-Blindness

Three to four per cent of all men and about 0.3 per cent of women are born color-blind. The absence of all appreciation of colors is very rare. In most cases, there is a lack of perception of red, green and/or blue.

Many color-blind people can develop their color sense. They can help themselves if they're willing to take the time and trouble.

My work with color-blindness began only incidentally when many years ago I was teaching a farsighted man to improve his near vision. It soon became apparent that he could not see colors well—a fact he seemed ashamed of and admitted reluctantly. The same problem came up in a number of subsequent male students, and I began to experiment with methods for developing better color sense along with better vision. There were many trials, many failures, later a few partial successes. Finally, a set of techniques proved effective for a number of young men whose color-blindness had been keeping them out of the Navy. All but one subsequently passed the Navy test.

The techniques are practical for self-instruction. If you are color-blind, there is a good chance that you can benefit from them.

Essentially, they add up to a double learning process. You will learn basic facts about colors and practice identifying, matching, making and sorting colors. You will also practice some of the basic elements of good vision and these will help to simplify and speed the color-learning process.

A first essential is to achieve relaxation. Tension affects your mind and memory and may interfere, too, with "sighting" of color. If previous attempts to learn color were futile, tension may have been a factor.

The basic relaxation techniques—sunning, palming and the long swing—will be of great help. Do them as described in Chapter III. When you practice mental imagery during palming, concentrate on colors, starting with those you know. If you can see yellow, visualize a yellow taxi. In your mind's eye, see houses, books, fruit, vegetables and other objects in yellow. See them in other colors you know. As you progress with your other practice and begin to recognize colors you've been blind to before, visualize them. And in your imagery, practice moving from color to color.

Mobility techniques are also important. Just as staring, poor shifting and slowness of sight blur letters for the near- and farsighted, so they may blur and distort color. The techniques for mobility given in Chapter IV will be of value to you. Do a lot of color counting as an aid to achieving mobility. Start with the colors you can see.

It will be helpful if you get six-inch rulers in colors. They're available in red, yellow, blue and green. Buy the colors you cannot now distinguish and use them in the ruler shift drill described in Chapter IV. You will be shifting on white lines. The white, which offers marked contrast, will help to bring in the colors for you.

You can also make a series of colored shifters instead of just the red one described in Chapter IV. Work first with the colors you can see, then, as you begin to get flashes of other colors, work with shifters in these newly seen colors.

Make your fusion devices (see Chapter v) in colors. For example, get a number of differently colored cords and change them (in the tubes) from day to day. Start with colors that you recognize easily. Work up to the more difficult ones. Make a colored fusion ring by alternating colored strips of tape. On your fusion yardstick, place colored thumbtacks along the working edge so that you can get a V or a channel with spots of color showing.

You can use colored tapes, changing them from time to time, to make the separation line between the two holes on the fusion plate. Use colored objects on the fusion cards. Have two groups of cards—one with colors that are easy for you, and another with difficult colors. Work from easy to difficult.

Comparison and contrast (see Chapter vii) are essential parts of your work. If you're looking at a color picture in a magazine, for example, don't try to "study" the colors. Instead, run your gaze across the background or around the white edges of the page and let the color "pop out" at you.

Good practice in using comparison and contrast is offered by the *Ishihara Plates for Testing Color Perception*, available in local libraries. Borrow the book when you first start your work and have a friend or relative go over it with you so you can note what you miss. (Later, at the end of the sixth week and at the end of the twelve weeks of work, you might like to go over it again to note your improvement.) While you have the plates, use them, too, for practice in comparison and contrast. For example, you will find some pink numbers on gray backgrounds which are on a black page. If you shift your gaze around the black, then around the edges of the gray square, then back and forth across the square, you will begin to get "flashes" of the pink color.

Many, if not most, color-blind people have other vision loss. If you are near- or farsighted, it will be helpful to add one accommodation technique from Chapter vi to your work each week. If you are nearsighted, practice for distance;

if you are farsighted, use the accommodation technique to help improve close point vision.

A good deal of your practice will be with water colors. Buy an inexpensive water color set and have a friend label the primary colors of red, yellow and blue.

Begin by making a daub of red, roughly one by one and a half inches in size, at the top and to the left of a sheet of white paper. Alongside the red, make equal-sized daubs of yellow and blue. Label these.

By combining two prime colors, you get a secondary color. Below the three daubs you have just made, write the words "secondary colors." Directly underneath and in the center, daub a bit of red and place an equal amount of yellow on top of the red. If the mixture has been equal, you will get the secondary color of orange. To the left of this, place another daub of red and add yellow, this time in greater quantity to get yellow-orange. To the right, place another daub of red and add to it less yellow to get red-orange. Label all three.

In the center of the next row, daub some yellow and place an equal amount of blue on top of it and the combination will be green. To the left of this, daub another bit of yellow and add to it less blue to get yellow-green. To the right, place another daub of yellow and add more blue for blue-green. Label all these.

Below this, center another daub of red, add an equal amount of blue, and you'll get purple or lavender. To the left, place another daub of red, add a lesser amount of blue, and you will have red-purple. To the right on another daub of red add more blue to get blue-purple. Label all of these, too.

Now on this one sheet you have the three primary colors and all of the secondary colors that can be made with them.

Later, you can go on to mix the three primes together to get brown, a tertiary color. You can also experiment with intensities. By adding more water to your yellow pigment, for example, you can make pale yellow. By adding less water you can make deep yellow. With more water added to red, you can make pale pink. With less water, you can make a heavy, rich red. With more water added to blue, you can make a pale, or baby blue. With less water, you get a deep blue.

Secondaries and tertiaries also have intensities of color. For example, purple may range in intensity from faint lilac to deep purple. Although black and white are not considered to be colors, there are intensities of black. If there is a black pigment in your paintbox, you can try adding enough water to it until you make it gray.

Have a friend check to make certain you're getting your colors and intensities right and also to measure your improvement from time to time.

After some practice, you can add another helpful drill. Everytime you use a different primary color, or make a different secondary or tertiary color, place a daub of it on a small sheet of paper.

Then, you can mix up the papers and try to label the colors. Have your friend check this. Do not be discouraged if at first you make many errors. The thing to watch for is the improvement that comes week after week.

Matching colors is the next important technique. Cut out various colors from magazine ads. You'll want two circles of each color, each circle the size of perhaps a quarter or even slightly smaller. Have your friend label the colors on the back of the circles. You'll be able to find all the prime colors, and all the secondaries and even all the tertiaries in various shades.

Keep all the reds in one envelope, the greens in another, the blues in another, etc. Label each envelope.

Start with an easy color—one that you can see relatively well. Let's say, it's blue. Take all of the colored circles out of the envelope marked "blue" and spread them out on the table before you. You should have about twenty pairs of blues in various tints. Match the pairs of each tint. Do the same with all the other colors.

You can and should do the same practice drill using pieces of colored cloth and yarn.

In all your color work, stop whenever you become fatigued. Rest yourself by sunning, palming, or just by letting your glance travel across a black cloth or black paper.

You can use the same paper circles and pieces of yarn and cloth in another drill—this time, arranging them in order of intensity. Start at the left side of the table with the lightest circle of a particular color and arrange the others in a row toward the right in the order of increasing intensity until you end with the most intense.

With the twelve-week program that follows, you will make a basic start in improving your color sense. At the end of that time, measure improvement by trying the Ishihara plates again.

If you can distinguish some colors that you could not distinguish before, you can stop working with these and concentrate on the colors that still bother you. As you continue your work, use the same drills and techniques. Keep practicing the sunning, palming, fusion and other drills for good vision as well as the color matching and sorting and other color-learning drills.

BASIC TWELVE-WEEK PROGRAM FOR COLOR-BLINDNESS

Every day, every week:

1. If you've been wearing glasses, remove them when you are doing the drills. Go without them as much as you can at other times—but never to the point of fatigue. Increase your "without glasses" time progressively from week to week.

2. Do the basic relaxation drills (see Chap iii).
   a. Sunning: 3-5 minutes at a time, 5 to 7 times.
   b. Palming: 3-5 minutes at a time, 5 to 7 times.
   c. Long swing: 2 minutes.
   d. Short swing, 1 or 2: 2 minutes total.
3. Count objects and colors (see Chapter iv) in free moments.
4. Practice vertical shifting (see Chapter iv): whenever possible.
5. If you are nearsighted: one near to far technique (see Chapter vi). Work as directed for nearsights. Change the techniques from day to day for variety.
   If you are farsighted: one far to near technique and some reading (see Chapters vi and viii). Work as directed for farsights. Change the techniques from day to day for variety.

Also each week:

1. See a technicolor movie.

IN ADDITION
Practice each day during the

FIRST WEEK

1. Cord fusion (Chap. v): 2-5 minutes.
(*Note:* Check yourself during this first week by going through a copy of Ishihara borrowed from your local library. Have a friend go over the plates with you. Note which ones you miss so you can check again for progress at the end of the sixth and twelfth weeks.)

SECOND WEEK

1. Work with water colors, making the "primes" of red, yellow and blue: 2-5 minutes.
2. Ring fusion (Chap. v)—put colored tapes on your ring: 2-5 minutes.

THIRD WEEK

1. Water color secondaries: 5-10 minutes.
2. Yardstick fusion (Chap. v): 2-4 minutes.

FOURTH WEEK

1. Water color (a) primes: 5 minutes; (b) secondaries: 5-10 minutes.
2. Christmas tree lights (Chap. IV): 3-6 minutes.
3. Colored shifters (Chap. IV): 2-6 minutes.
4. Cord fusion (Chap. v): with colored cord: 2-4 minutes.
5. Ring fusion (Chap. v): 2-4 minutes.

FIFTH WEEK

1. Match colored circles: 10-20 minutes.
2. Plate fusion (Chap. v): 2 minutes.
3. Yardstick fusion (Chap. v): 2-4 minutes.

SIXTH WEEK

1. Water color primes and secondaries: 15-20 minutes.
2. Colored shifters (Chap. IV): 2-6 minutes.
3. Cord fusion (Chap. v): 2-4 minutes.
4. Yardstick fusion to colored objects in distance, such as books in bookcase (Chap. VI): 3-4 minutes.
5. Try Ishihara again. (See how many more you can get.)

SEVENTH WEEK

1. Match colored circles. Place them in order of intensity of color (light to dark): 15-20 minutes.
2. Colored shifters (Chap. IV): 2-6 minutes.
3. Cord fusion (Chap. v): 2-4 minutes.
4. Ring fusion (Chap. v): 2-4 minutes.

EIGHTH WEEK

1. Water colors, light to dark, primes and secondaries: 15-20 minutes.

2. Colored shifters (Chap. IV): 2-6 minutes.
3. Christmas tree lights and mirror (Chap. IV): 3-6 minutes.
4. Yardstick fusion (Chap. V): 2-4 minutes.
5. Plate fusion (Chap. V): 2-4 minutes.

NINTH WEEK

1. Match colored circles and place them in order of intensity. (Colored circles should now be cut down to size of dime.): 15-20 minutes.
2. Match yarns or pieces of cloth: 5-10 minutes.
3. Colored shifters (Chap. IV): 2-6 minutes.
4. Ring fusion (Chap. V): 2-4 minutes.
5. Fusion cards (Chap. V): 2-4 minutes.

TENTH WEEK

1. Water colors light to dark, primes, secondaries and tertiaries: 15-25 minutes.
2. Match yarns and pieces of cloth: 5-10 minutes.
3. Christmas tree lights and mirror (Chap. IV): 3-6 minutes.
4. Fusion cards (Chap. V): 1-3 minutes.
5. Cord fusion (Chap. V): 2-4 minutes.

ELEVENTH WEEK

1. Match colored cloth or yarns. Then place them, color by color, in order of their intensity: 15-25 minutes.
2. Colored shifters (Chap. IV): 2-6 minutes.
3. Christmas tree lights and mirror (Chap. IV): 3-6 minutes.
4. Ring fusion (Chap. V): 2-4 minutes.
5. Plate fusion (Chap. V): 2-4 minutes.

TWELFTH WEEK

1. Water colors (small *dots* of primes, secondaries and tertiaries in order of their intensity): 15-25 minutes.

2. Colored shifters (Chap. IV): 2-6 minutes.
3. Try Ishihara again.
4. Cord fusion (Chap. v): 2-5 minutes.
5. Fusion cards (Chap. v): 2-4 minutes.

CASE HISTORY

A. M. came for lessons because his color-blindness had kept him out of the Navy. He also had a doctor's diagnosis of myopia although it was of such a minor degree that he passed the Navy test for distance which, at that time, required 20/40 vision but missed all but two of the Navy's color plates.

In the first lesson, he was taught the basic relaxation techniques. We started some mobility drills, cord fusion and letter boards, too.

Then with three water colors—red, yellow and blue—I made up the primary and secondary color sheet, explaining each step and adding that all colors in the Ishihara plates could be made with the three primes.

He took the sheet home with him. For homework, he was to mix colors every day, date them and bring them to me on the next lesson. Like almost all of the boys who came to me during World War II, he worked faithfully.

On his second lesson he could see several more of the Ishihara plates. I introduced him to the lighter and deeper shades of primes and secondaries. And in this lesson we began to work more intensively with fusion techniques. A red fusion cord was substituted for the white one, and he got occasional flashes of "a color I've never seen before." He worked well with yardstick fusion. And after some practice I had him point the yardstick at an Oriental rug on the floor and pick out colors as they appeared in the illusionary channel between two yardsticks. The colors, he said, seemed brighter. He called many correctly.

He kept up his homework practice of mixing colors along

with the relaxation, mobility and fusion drills, and on his next lesson he got two more of the Ishihara plates.

Then I asked him to have a friend help him cut out colors in magazine advertisements and to start matching them. He still continued mixing colors and dating them and bringing them in.

In succeeding lessons, we added accommodation drills to help his nearsightedness. He continued the other practice and got his girl friend to go window-shopping with him. She was sympathetic with his desire to enlist in the Navy and would correct him patiently when he miscalled a color. Her sympathy was so complete that she *never* laughed at him when he made an error.

By the time he had his eighth lesson he was identifying correctly the color of 80 per cent of the books on the shelves in my office and was calling correctly 50 percent of the numbers on the Ishihara plates.

He was still mixing secondary colors. I then added tints, hues and tertiaries. He persistently practiced mixing and labeling them.

On his sixteenth lesson he named all of the Ishihara plates correctly.

There were four more weekly lessons and he practiced his homework diligently.

Color-blind people learn to tell traffic light signals by memorizing the positions of red, amber and green. Just before we concluded the last lesson, I suddenly asked him, "Which color, red or green, is at the top on a traffic light?" He looked blank for a moment, then told me, adding, "I had begun to forget the positions now that I can tell the colors and don't have to think which is where."

The following week he passed his test for the Navy.

Chapter XVI

Step-by-Step for Glaucoma

If your sight has been impaired by glaucoma, the techniques of visual retraining may be of great value.

In glaucoma, the channels that normally drain eye fluid are blocked, and, as a result, pressure within the eye is raised. Periods of blurred vision are experienced. Headaches may occur, especially in the dark or upon awakening. There is a progressive loss of clear vision at the close point and side vision is diminished, too.

The cause of glaucoma is still not understood. It has been suggested that possibly advanced age and hardening of the arteries may be predisposing factors. Some recent medical investigations have linked the disease with emotional problems. In one recent study, attacks of glaucoma were found to coincide frequently with emotional upsets. Case histories of many of the glaucoma victims with whom I've worked tend to indicate, too, that emotional shock may have played a part in causing the trouble.

Almost all of my glaucoma students were under physician's care. Visual retraining need not be, and I have never allowed it to be, a substitute for medical treatment and supervision. Most of my students were using medication prescribed for them by their physicians when they first came for lessons—and continued to use it. In many cases, they were able to discontinue medication upon successful completion of visual retraining, but they were always advised to do so only after re-examination by their physician and upon his recommendation.

If you have glaucoma—and this should not be a matter of guesswork but should be something you know as the result of expert medical diagnosis—the program offered in this chapter is not a panacea, yet there is a good chance that you will find it helpful in improving your vision.

It makes use of many of the basic techniques employed in helping to overcome other types of sight loss. There are also some special techniques which have proved to be particularly useful for people with glaucoma.

SPECIAL TECHNIQUES

As with all other type of vision difficulty, relaxation is essential. If anything, it is even more essential and helpful for people with glaucoma. In the last few years, since I have been placing increasing emphasis on sunning, one of the basic relaxation techniques, I have noted that improvement has come more rapidly.

Some years ago, I was told the story of a doctor with early glaucoma who consulted an eye specialist and received what he thought was an unusual prescription. "Just try going out on your lawn several times every sunny day," the specialist advised. "Lie down, close your eyes, relax. Let the sun shine on your closed eyelids and gently and easily turn your head from side to side. Do this for just about two minutes at a time." The doctor, who is still working at his profession, has had no further trouble with glaucoma.

Sunning has a relaxing effect on the eyes—and the whole body. In addition to the sunning techniques given in Chapter III, two additional ones will be helpful for you.

Technique 1: Set up your light in front of the chair you regularly use for sunning, at the usual distance. Place a second chair alongside the sunning lamp. You will need two squares of 18" x 18" cardboard, one red and one blue. For the red one, you can use the back of your domino wheel. Turn on your sunning light and take two minutes of the white light on your closed lids in your regular chair. Then, move over to the chair next to the sunning lamp, pick up the red cardboard, hold it out with both hands in front of your eyes and move it until you have it at the proper angle so that it picks up the light from the sunning lamp and reflects it onto your eyelids. Keep your eyes closed as you take five minutes of this reflected red glow. Repeat with the blue card, also for five minutes.

Technique 2: For this, you will need a yellow 18″ x 18″ board in addition to the red. Start by taking two minutes of white light, then five minutes of red glow, as above. Follow this with five minutes of yellow glow from the third cardboard and finish with five minutes of white light back in the original chair.

Light is stimulating to the vision. Some doctors recently have been urging glaucoma patients to stop wearing dark glasses as much as possible and to sleep with a small light on nearby. Both measures, I believe, are helpful.

Do the mobility techniques called for in your twelve-week program as described in Chapter IV. Use yardstick, rather than ruler, shifting since the yardstick's length will help widen your field of vision.

For another good vision-widening drill seat yourself in an armchair, with your elbows supported on the chair's arms and your open hands held about a foot in front of your eyes. Your hands should be as far apart as you can hold them and still see both while looking straight ahead. With a head motion, look from one hand to the other. Go back and forth four times. Repeat with your eyes closed, remembering the position of your hands. Then do this four times again with the eyes open.

Now, move your hands apart another inch and repeat the drill. When you've finished, you should be able to look straight ahead of you and be aware of both hands at this increased distance. In other words, you should have widened at least temporarily your field of vision by an inch. If you have not been able to do so, repeat the drill.

Then, go on, progressively increasing the distance between the hands from day to day until you reach the point where, with your hands almost even with your ears, you can look ahead and still be aware of both.

OTHER WORK

The rest of the work you will do involves techniques useful in other types of visual problems. You will palm and use mental imagery and do the long swing for relaxation, too. You will use the fusion and accommodation drills, all as described in the opening chapters of the book. In doing the letter board work, if you can see clearly the letters in letter board No. 2 at ten feet, you can work it and do not need to make up letter board No. 1. If you cannot, make up No. 1 and use it until you can see letter board No. 2 at ten feet.

To improve your vision at the close point, you will do much of your practice by reading. Helpful suggestions on how to do this will be found in Chapter VIII.

The twelve-week program which follows will give you a proper balance of techniques. You should find it practical in terms of time. If there are days when you cannot get in all the practice called for, sunning and palming come first.

On the basis of the experience of others with glaucoma, at the end of the twelve weeks, your doctor should find at least a small drop in pressure within your eyes. You should be able to see more clearly at all distances and your field of vision should have widened considerably. Best of all, you should have lost some, and possibly all, of your fear of glaucoma and of possible blindness.

It will probably be necessary for you to continue with the

sunning, palming and fusion work indefinitely. But if a half-hour or so daily of this practice holds your sight, if your doctor continues in his regular checkups to find that your glaucoma remains under control, it is, as you will agree, a small price to pay.

After you've completed the twelve-week program, you can expect to make further gains if you continue with all of the drills. You can use the work given in the twelve weeks as a basis for developing a program of your own. You will probably like certain techniques more than others and may have found some that seem to bring you more benefit. You can build your program around these techniques. Be sure, however, to include sunning and palming. Be sure, too, that your program is balanced and contains one or more techniques for relaxation, mobility and centralization, for fusion and for accommodation.

When your tension is gone, according to your doctor, and your sight has improved although still not normal, you can use the work in Chapter xi or xii, according to whether you were originally near- or farsighted.

BASIC TWELVE-WEEK PROGRAM FOR GLAUCOMA

Every day, every week:

1. Leave your glasses off when doing the drills. Go without them as much as you can at other times—but never to the point of fatigue. Increase your "without glasses" time progressively from week to week.
2. Do the basic relaxation drills (see Chapter iii)
   a. Sunning: 4 minutes at a time, 6 to 8 times.
   b. Palming with visual imagery: 2 minutes at a time, 6 to 8 times a day.
   c. Long swing: 2 minutes.
   d. Short swings: one or two: 2 minutes total.

3. Count objects and colors in free moments (see Chapter iv) as much as possible.
4. Practice vertical shifting whenever possible (see Chapter iv).
5. Practice with the red shifter (see Chapter iv) whenever possible.

Also each week:

1. See a movie if it does not tire you and follow suggestions in Chapter x.

IN ADDITION
Practice each day during the

FIRST WEEK

1. Letter board (Chap. vi): 5-8 minutes.
2. Reading (Chap. viii): newspaper headlines or magazine advertisements or book reading: 10-20 minutes.
3. Cord fusion (Chap. v): 1-3 minutes.

SECOND WEEK

1. Domino wheels (Chap. vi): 2-4 minutes.
2. Colored glow sunning, technique 1 (Chap. xvi): 12 minutes.
3. Reading (Chap. viii): newspaper headlines, magazine advertisements or book: 10-20 minutes.
4. Ring shift (Chap. iv): 1-3 minutes.
5. Cord fusion (Chap. v): 2-4 minutes.

THIRD WEEK

1. Letter board (Chap. vi): 5-8 minutes.
2. Solitaire (Chap. iv): 1 game with each eye; one with both together.
3. Colored glow sunning, technique 2 (Chap. xvi): 17 minutes.

4. Reading (Chap. vm): newspaper headlines, magazine advertisements or book: 15-30 minutes.
5. Ring shift (Chap. iv): 1-3 minutes.
6. Ring fusion (Chap. v): 1-3 minutes.
7. Cord fusion (Chap. v): 2-4 minutes.

FOURTH WEEK

1. Playing card drill (Chap. vi): 5-12 minutes.
2. Colored glow sunning, technique 1 (Chap. xvi): 12 minutes.
3. Toss ball (Chap. iv): 2-4 minutes.
4. Yardstick shift (Chap. iv): 1-3 minutes.
5. Reading (Chap. vm): Gettysburg Address (see p. 111) or larger print: 15 minutes.
6. Boat fusion (Chap. v): 1-2 minutes.
7. Cord fusion (Chap. v): 2-5 minutes.

FIFTH WEEK

1. Letter board (Chap. vi): with each eye: 8-12 minutes total time.
2. Colored glow sunning, technique 2 (Chap. xvi): 17 minutes.
3. Solitaire (Chap. iv): with both eyes, 1 game.
4. Reading (Chap. vm): Gettysburg Address (see p. 111) or larger print: 15-30 minutes.
5. Yardstick shift (Chap. iv): 1-3 minutes.
6. Ruler fusion (Chap. v): 1-2 minutes.
7. Cord fusion (Chap. vm): 2-4 minutes.

SIXTH WEEK

1. Playing card drill (Chap. vi): with each eye: 4-10 minutes total time.
2. Colored glow sunning, technique 1 (Chap. xvi): 12 minutes.
3. Domino wheels (Chap. vi): 2-4 minutes.

4. Reading (Chap. viii): 15-30 minutes.
5. Fusion plate (Chap. v): 1-3 minutes.
6. Ring shift (Chap. iv): 1-3 minutes.
7. Toss ball (Chap. iv): 1-3 minutes.
8. Cord fusion (Chap. v): 2-4 minutes.

SEVENTH WEEK

1. Jumbled numbers (Chap. vi): with each eye separately, 4-6 minutes total time.
2. Jumbled letters (Chap. vi): with both eyes together: 2-5 minutes.
3. Yardstick shift (Chap. iv): 2-4 minutes.
4. Colored glow sunning, technique 2 (Chap. xvi): 17 minutes.
5. Reading (Chap. viii): 15-40 minutes.
6. Ring fusion (Chap. v): 2-4 minutes.

EIGHTH WEEK

1. Letter board (Chap. vi): with each eye: 8-15 minutes total time.
2. Playing card drill (Chap. vi): with both eyes together: 5-8 minutes.
3. Colored glow sunning, technique 1 (Chap. xvi): 12 minutes.
4. Reading (Chap. viii): with each eye: 2-5 minutes.
5. Ring shift (Chap. iv): 1-3 minutes.
6. Boat fusion (Chap. v): 1-3 minutes.
7. Cord fusion (Chap. v): 2-4 minutes.

NINTH WEEK

1. Jumbled letters (Chap. vi): with each eye: 4-10 minutes total time.
   Jumbled numbers (Chap. vi): with both eyes together: 2-5 minutes.

2. Domino wheels (Chap. vi): 2-4 minutes.
3. Colored glow sunning, technique 2 (Chap. xvi): 17 minutes.
4. Yardstick shift (Chap. iv): 1-3 minutes.
5. Reading (Chap. viii): with each eye: 3-5 minutes; with both eyes: 10-30 minutes.
6. Plate fusion (Chap. v): 1-3 minutes.
7. Cord fusion (Chap. v): 2-4 minutes.

TENTH WEEK

1. Letter board (Chap. vi): with each eye: 8-15 minutes total time.
2. Solitaire (Chap. iv): with both eyes: 10-15 minutes.
3. Toss ball (Chap. iv): 2-4 minutes.
4. Colored glow sunning, technique 1 (Chap. xvi): 12 minutes.
5. Reading (Chap. viii): with both eyes together, 15-40 minutes.
6. Boat fusion (Chap. v): 1-3 minutes.
7. Yardstick fusion (Chap. v): 2-4 minutes.

ELEVENTH WEEK

1. Playing card drill (Chap. vi): with each eye: 8-15 minutes total time.
2. Letter board (Chap. vi): with both eyes together: 5-8 minutes.
3. Yardstick shifting (Chap. iv): 1-3 minutes.
4. Colored glow sunning, technique 2 (Chap. xvi): 17 minutes.
5. Reading (Chap. viii): with each eye: 2-5 minutes; with both eyes together: 15-40 minutes.
6. Card fusion (Chap. v): 1-3 minutes.
7. Ring fusion (Chap. v): 1-3 minutes.
8. Cord fusion (Chap. v): 2-4 minutes.

TWELFTH WEEK

1. Jumbled letters (Chap. vi): with one eye: 2-4 minutes.
2. Jumbled numbers (Chap. vi): with the other eye: 2-4 minutes.
3. Letter board (Chap. vi): with both eyes together: 5-8 minutes.
4. Colored glow sunning technique 1 (Chap. xvi): 12 minutes.
5. Reading (Chap. viii): with each eye for 2-5 minutes; with both eyes together: 15-45 minutes.
6. Ring shift (Chap. iv): 1-3 minutes.
7. Card fusion (Chap. v): 1-2 minutes.
8. Boat fusion (Chap. v): 1-2 minutes.
9. Plate fusion (Chap. v): 1-2 minutes.

CASE HISTORIES

Mr. R., a man of about sixty, had had glaucoma for eight years. According to his doctor, he had a visual acuity of 20/400 in his left eye and 20/70 in the right. Surgery had been performed on the left eye, but not on the right. The doctor had recently told him that cataract was developing in the left eye. He had started to wear reading glasses fourteen years before and had worn bifocals for ten years. He had great reading difficulty with or without glasses.

He said that he was using drops in both eyes. He asked me if he should discontinue them. The answer was, "No, I never interfere with a doctor's treatment."

During his first lessons, he was taught the sunning, palming and mobility drills. He did board 9 from about ten feet with both eyes together. The long swing was stressed as a means of gaining greater field. He was also shown how to shift along a yardstick and to work the playing card drill.

The fusion cord was very difficult, but he finally mastered it out to about five feet. He said that his wife would help him with the cord.

During the second lesson, a week later, he did board 10 from a foot farther out. He was given an eye patch and was able to see some of board No. 1 at about six feet with his left eye. He was instructed to swing his head back and forth across the rows of letters, calling any that he saw. With his right eye, he saw some of board No. 11 at the same distance he had seen board 10 with both eyes. Fusion was better and he was given a ring for practice.

At the beginning of his next lesson, he said that he had seen a definite improvement in acuity and area. We began colored glow sunning, and he was very diligent about this at home.

When he came for his sixth lesson, he said that he had had his regular checkup by his eye specialist and he was vastly cheered that the tension was down four points in his right eye and two in his left eye.

A few weeks later, he did board 14 at approximately fifteen feet and board 6 at about six feet with his left eye. Advanced fusion techniques and more widening drills were added, and he said he was going to ask his doctor to check his field at his next visit.

I was away on vacation during the next week. When he came after that for his next lesson, he reported that the tension was down three more points in the right eye, and two in the left eye, and the doctor had also said that his cataract was showing no increase and that he had a greater field of vision.

He said that he wanted to try to take the driver's test without glasses, but I asked him to wait.

His vision showed a steady increase during the next eighteen lessons, spaced over a year. At the end of that time, he passed his driver's test with 20/20 vision in the right eye and 20/100 in the left eye. His report from the doctor showed normal tension in the right eye and only two points above normal in the left eye.

He continued his lessons until we reached what seemed to

be his potential in the operated eye, and the doctor said there was no cataract and the tension was normal. In the final lessons, we concentrated on reading distance. He now reads newspapers, telephone books and menus without glasses.

Mr. R. G., a lawyer, came to me with the doctor's diagnosis of glaucoma. He said that he had been under extreme tension for some time and would continue to be because of a domestic problem and several important and difficult legal cases and wouldn't have too much time to practice. He had worn reading glasses for several years. Recently his doctor had said that his distance sight had dropped, too. He had only a slight loss of visual field.

In the first lesson, we worked on relaxation and mobility techniques and finished with a few accommodation drills. He did manage to do a good bit of home practice and showed improvement and he was taught some reading techniques. He was also shown how to practice to widen his field.

In the third lesson, both his distance and close point vision showed improvement. Again basic relaxation techniques were stressed. He decided to take up bridge and golf again and thought he could play both games without glasses.

The following week he read the smallest type on graduated print sets. I asked him to continue his homework and wait two weeks for the next lesson.

In the interim, he went back to his doctor for a regular checkup on tension. It was down four points.

In the following three months, his tension, according to his doctor, became normal. He still suns and palms. His distance sight is excellent and he has a weaker pair of glasses for reading.

Mrs. L. R. had had glaucoma for several years and had had two operations. Her sight was very poor and she could read only newspaper headlines and see only very large letters, three or four inches high, a few feet away.

She was given the basic relaxation drills and was told to do lots of sunning and palming.

She reported the following week that she was seeing a clock in her living room more clearly than she had in a long time. She also said that she was a little more sure of herself when walking.

On the second lesson she did a letter board and was taught some of the widening drills.

She added playing cards and dominoes to her homework. She liked the red shifter and used it several times every day.

At the end of two months she was playing solitaire and doing the domino wheel each day at home.

While her sight is not normal she has increased it greatly. She rarely feels eye discomfort now. She still continues her sunning and palming, accommodation and other drills. She likes them, she says, and while she feels no urgent need to improve her vision still more, she is slowly increasing her acuity working by herself.

Chapter XVII

Step-by-Step for Cataract

Cataract is not a growth but rather a gradual loss of transparency in the lens of the eye. The word itself is derived from the Greek word meaning waterfall and it may have been applied to the eye problem because, as the lens loses transparency, the vision loss may seem like what one would expect if something were dropping in front of the eye.

The degree of vision loss, of course, depends upon the location and extent of the opacity. When cataracts are far-advanced and diffuse, vision may be reduced until only light perception remains. In the early stages of cataracts, near-sightedness often develops so that a patient who previously has been farsighted may discover that he can read without his glasses. There is even a term used to describe this—"second sight."

During the development of a cataract, frequent changes of glasses help to maintain useful vision for as long as possible. With considerable impairment of vision, surgical removal of the lens is often performed.

Over the last ten years, I have seen many people with cataracts helped to a rewarding extent by vision retraining techniques. Most of them have remained under medical supervision while using the techniques and have returned for periodic checkups to their physicians. Some, in whom the need for surgery had seemed imminent, were able to avert the operation and are now benefiting from glasses.

Some have been able to go beyond this and dispense with glasses.

With a few modifications, the techniques used have been the same as those employed to help people with other eye problems. Why should these methods work for people with cataract?

I am frank to say that I do not know the whole answer. Most of us may not make full use of our visual capacity because of poor seeing habits. People with cataracts are no exception. If the only result when a person with cataract undertook visual retraining was some improvement in vision, it could be explained on the grounds of better use of remaining visual capacity. But, in many cases, re-examination by physicians after some weeks or months of visual work has shown reductions in size and severity of opacities.

If you have a cataract problem, there is a good chance that you will derive benefits from the program given in this chapter. It is not offered as a panacea but as a worthwhile help.

It calls for the use of a wide variety of techniques, all described in Chapters III through VII, aimed at achieving relaxation and building up proper habits of seeing. Except as otherwise noted here, you can practice all of them when called for in the step-by-step program, exactly as described in the earlier chapters.

The basic relaxation techniques of sunning and palming have proved especially helpful for people with cataract. You will spend much more time on them than do people with most other types of vision loss.

If you are bothered by light, it will be advisable to begin your sunning work either at a little greater distance from the lamp than suggested in Chapter III or you may wish to use a smaller bulb. You can work with one as small as 40 watts. Gradually, as your sensitivity to light decreases, you will be able to take the light as directed in Chapter III.

An additional sunning technique has proved to be valuable for many people with cataract. Have your regular light set up in front of the chair you usually use for sunning, at the regular distance. Place a second chair alongside the sunning lamp. You will need two squares of cardboard 18″ x 18″, one red and one yellow. For the red one, you can use the back of your large domino wheel.

Begin by turning on your sunning light to get two minutes of the white light on your closed lids. Then move over to the chair next to the sunning lamp, hold the red cardboard out with both hands in front of your eyes and move it until you find the proper angle at which it picks up the light from the lamp and reflects it back onto your closed eyes. With your eyes closed, take five minutes of this reflected red glow. Then move back to the first chair and take two minutes more of white light. After this, move back to the chair beside the light and repeat the reflected glow technique for five minutes, this time using the yellow cardboard. Finally, palm for one minute.

In my experience, red seems to have a stimulating effect while yellow has a relaxing one. The alternate stimulation and relaxation seems to be particularly effective in improving the sight of people with cataract.

Walking to and from a mirror is an important aid in cataracts. It provides a change of focus and accommodation. It should be done with music.

Stand four feet away from a mirror, then walk directly toward it until you are only a foot away, watching your face in the mirror all the time. Walk backward now, away from the mirror, still watching your face and return to the original four-foot mark. Repeat this for one minute or longer, as called for in the step-by-step program.

The mirror walk is also done with one eye at a time. Cover one eye with the cupped palm of your hand and let the eye remain open underneath. Turn your nose one-half inch in the direction of the uncovered eye. Then, looking in toward your face in the mirror, walk to and from as above. Repeat, covering the other eye, turning the face the other way.

If you are like most of the people with cataract with whom I've worked, you will have days when you see better than others—primarily because of the particular light conditions. (Many people with cataracts like overcast days rather than sunny ones.) Therefore, some days, in your practice with the letter board and other drills, you may feel that you are making no progress, maybe even going backward. You should not be discouraged. As you keep practicing, you will be able to use more and more light on your work and there will be less and less of a tendency for variations in visual acuity from day to day.

People with cataract need serenity and harmony to tide them over their fluctuations of sight. They have told me that emotional upsets cause their vision to become more foggy, that a cold has the same effect upon them. Some have volunteered that they experience tremendous loss of sight when they are very tired. Many people with cataract have told me that they first noticed their loss of sight during an emotional crisis. Some of them have told me that they have a continuation of crises so that they are always tense.

Most cataract cases for this reason need to do a tremendous amount of visual imagery which is pleasant and happy.

Try to regulate your thinking and your visual imagery to encompass clarity of thought and memory. It is even more important than the physical work connected with mobility and fusion which should be part of your practice.

It's important that you never strain—never make any tremendous effort to see—and this is particularly true in the accommodation work. Work slowly, easily, seeking greater clarity rather than greater distance. If, for example, you can see the letter board clearly at a distance of four feet but poorly at five feet, you should not strain to see it at the farther distance. Concentrate on attaining ever-increasing clarity and speed at the shorter distance. Never fear that you will not see at greater distances. You will, almost automatically, as you improve the clarity at the shorter distances.

In doing the letter board work, if you can see clearly the letters in letter board No. 2 at ten feet, you can work it and do not need to make up letter board No. 1. Otherwise, start with No. 1, using it until you can see No. 2 at ten feet.

Some of the time in your letter board practice, you can use this method to help gently extend your sight: Set up a card table about ten feet from a door mirror. Place a string of five lighted Christmas tree lights at the far edge of the card table. Set your distant letter board halfway between table and mirror, just a little lower than the lights so you can still see the latter in the mirror.

Pick up a letter in your hand, look from the first light to the fifth light with a head motion, then look at the reflections of the same lights in the mirror, again moving from one to the other with a head motion, then glance at the distant letter board and find the letter. You can vary the technique by choosing different lights, working from 2 to 4 or 3 to 5 or 2 to 5.

In all practice, avoid fatigue. Never work any drill when you feel tired. Always stop short of fatigue. If you begin to feel even slightly tired in the midst of a drill, stop and do some sunning and palming before going on.

It's essential to remember that the habits of good vision you are trying to establish in the formal drills must be carried over into the whole pattern of your daily life. This is true for all people with impaired vision and has been mentioned before. People with cataract, perhaps because they tend to be older and a little more set in their ways, sometimes have more difficulty in remembering to practice good vision techniques throughout the day until they become habits.

At the end of the twelve weeks' work you will probably notice a definite improvement in your vision. Frequently, people who wore glasses when they started, but volunteered they didn't really know why since their vision seemed no better with them on or off, find a distinct difference at the end of the twelve weeks. They are not at the point where they can dispense with glasses—but their glasses now help them to see better.

This does not necessarily mean the end of the road. Work should be continued until the full potential of sight is developed—and for some this may mean, at the end of a year or longer, excellent sight at all distances without glasses.

I suggest, for all people with cataract, a medical re-examination at the end of the first twelve weeks. Frequently, the physician finds not only better vision but an arrest in the cataract's progress and, in some cases, an actual improvement. Even the discovery that the cataract is no longer progressing is a great morale-booster and incentive to continue work.

In further work, you can use the twelve weeks' program as a basis. To these techniques, you can add more of the accommodation drills described in Chapter vi: If you were originally nearsighted, work from near to far. If you were originally farsighted, practice accommodation from far to near. You will also be able to go into more advanced fusion work, including the card fusion described in Chapter v.

When your doctor tells you that you no longer have cataract but your vision is still not normal, you can do the twelve weeks' work in Chapter xi or xii, depending on whether you are nearsighted or farsighted.

BASIC TWELVE-WEEK PROGRAM
FOR CATARACT

Every day, every week:

1. Leave your glasses off when doing the drills. Go without them as much as possible at other times—but never to the point of fatigue. Increase your "without glasses" time progressively from week to week.
2. Do the basic relaxation drills (see Chapter III)
   a. Sunning: 6 sessions of 4 minutes each, or equivalent.
   b. Palming with visual imagery: 6 sessions of 4 minutes each, or equivalent.
   c. Long swing: morning and evening: 2 minutes each time.
   d. Short swings: one or more: 2 minutes total.
3. Count objects and colors (see Chapter IV): in free moments.
4. Practice vertical shifting (see Chapter IV): whenever possible.
5. Toss ball (see Chapter IV): 2-4 minutes.
6. Walk to and from mirror (Chapter XVII): 2 minutes.

Also each week:

1. See a movie if it does not tire you.
2. Practice colored glow sunning (Chap. XVII) two or three times, more often if possible.

IN ADDITION
Practice each day during the

FIRST WEEK

1. Letter board (Chap. VI): 6-8 minutes.
2. Alternate sunning and palming (Chap. III): 2 minutes.
3. Ruler shift (Chap. IV): 1-3 minutes.
4. Reading (Chap. VIII): newspaper headlines and advertisements: 5-10 minutes.
5. Cord fusion (Chap. V): 3-8 minutes.

SECOND WEEK

1. Reading (Chap. viii): smallest print you can do with ease, from newspaper headlines to very small print: 5-10 minutes.
2. Playing card drill (Chap. vi): 5-8 minutes.
3. Jumbled letters (Chap. v): 4-6 minutes.
4. Red shifter (Chap. iv): 2-5 minutes.
5. Cord fusion (Chap. v): 3-5 minutes.

THIRD WEEK

1. Jumbled numbers (Chap. vi): 5-6 minutes.
2. Reading (Chap. vi): smallest print you can do with ease, from newspaper headlines to very small print: 12-15 minutes.
3. Letter board (Chap. vi): 5-8 minutes.
4. Christmas tree lights (Chap. iv): 2-4 minutes.
5. Red shifter (Chap. iv): 1-3 minutes.
6. Ring shift (Chap. iv): 1-3 minutes.
7. Cord fusion (Chap. v): 3-5 minutes.

FOURTH WEEK

1. Jumbled letters (Chap. vi): 3-6 minutes.
2. Reading (Chap. viii): smallest print you can do with ease, from newspaper headlines to very small print: 15-20 minutes.
3. Domino wheels (Chap. vi): 2-3 minutes.
4. Solitaire (Chap. iv): with each eye (if sight good enough, otherwise with both eyes together): 10-20 minutes.

FIFTH WEEK

1. Reading (Chap. viii): smallest print you can do with ease, from newspaper headlines to very small print: 15-30 minutes.
2. Letter board (Chap. vi): 5-8 minutes.

3. Jumbled numbers (Chap. vi): 3-4 minutes.
4. Solitaire (Chap. iv): see previous week's directions.
5. Ruler shifter (Chap. iv): 1-3 minutes.
6. Christmas tree lights in mirror (Chap. iv): 4-8 minutes.
7. Cord fusion (Chap. v): 1-3 minutes.

SIXTH WEEK

1. Reading (Chap. viii): smallest print you can do with ease, from newspaper headlines to very small print: 15-40 minutes.
2. Letter board (Chap. vi): ½ with each eye if sight good enough: 8-16 minutes.
3. Jumbled numbers (Chap. vi): both eyes together: 2-5 minutes.
4. Christmas tree lights (Chap. iv): 4-6 minutes.
5. Yardstick fusion (Chap. v): 1-3 minutes.
6. Ring fusion (Chap. v): 1-3 minutes.

SEVENTH WEEK

1. Reading (Chap. viii): smallest print you can do with ease, from newspaper headlines to very small print: 15-40 minutes.
2. Jumbled letters (Chap. vi): 2-5 minutes.
3. Domino wheels (Chap. vi): 1-3 minutes.
4. Solitaire (Chap. iv): with each eye: 8-20 minutes total time.
5. Red shifter (Chap. iv): 1-3 minutes.
6. Yardstick shifting (Chap. iv): 1-3 minutes.
7. Cord fusion (Chap. v): 2-4 minutes.
8. Ring fusion (Chap. v): 1-3 minutes.

EIGHTH WEEK

1. Reading (Chap. viii): smallest print you can do with ease, from newspaper headlines to very small print: 20-50 minutes.

2. Christmas tree lights in mirror (Chap. III): each eye separately: 1-3 minutes; both eyes together: 2 minutes.
3. Jumbled numbers (Chap. VI): 2-5 minutes.
4. Domino wheels (Chap. VI): 2-5 minutes.
5. Yardstick fusion (Chap. VI): 1-3 minutes.
6. Plate fusion (Chap. V): 1-3 minutes.

NINTH WEEK

1. Reading (Chap. VIII): smallest print you can see with ease, from newspaper headlines to very small print: 20-50 minutes.
2. Reading, with each eye separately: 2-4 minutes.
3. Letter board (Chap. VI): both eyes together: 5-8 minutes.
4. Red shifter (Chap. VIII): 1-3 minutes.
5. Ring shift (Chap. IV): 3-4 minutes.
6. Cord fusion (Chap. V): 2-4 minutes.
7. Plate fusion (Chap. V): 1-3 minutes.

TENTH WEEK

1. Reading (Chap. VIII): smallest print you can do with ease, from newspaper headlines to very small print: 20-60 minutes.
2. Jumbled letters (Chap. VI): each eye separately: 2-6 minutes total time.
3. Playing card drill (Chap. VI): both eyes together: 8-12 minutes.
4. Yardstick shift (Chap. IV): 1-3 minutes.
5. Card fusion (Chap. V): 1-3 minutes.
6. Yardstick fusion (Chap. V): 1-3 minutes.

ELEVENTH WEEK

1. Reading (Chap. VIII): smallest print you can do with ease, from newspaper headlines to very small print: 20-60 minutes.

2. Christmas tree lights in mirror (Chap. IV): each eye separately: 3-6 minutes total time.
3. Letter board (Chap. VI): both eyes together: 5-8 minutes.
4. Ring shift (Chap. IV): 1-3 minutes.
5. Domino wheels (Chap. VI): 1-3 minutes.
6. Cord fusion (Chap. V): 1-3 minutes.
7. Card fusion (Chap. V): 1-3 minutes.

TWELFTH WEEK

1. Reading (Chap. VIII): smallest print you can do with ease, from newspaper headlines to very small print: 20-60 minutes.
2. Letter board (Chap. VI): with each eye separately: 8-10 minutes total.
3. Playing card drill (Chap. VI): 5-8 minutes.
4. Ring shift (Chap. IV): 1-3 minutes.
5. Yardstick shift (Chap. IV): 1-3 minutes.
6. Ring fusion (Chap. V): 2-4 minutes.
7. Card fusion (Chap. V): 1-3 minutes.

CASE HISTORIES

While I have had successful cataract cases whose ages varied from six to ninety-two, I shall choose cases between these extremes for examples.

Mr. F. was about seventy when he started his lessons. One eye, according to his doctor, was a "dead eye" from cataract—to be forgotten. Sight was so poor that the doctor gave him no measure of acuity. The other eye, also cataractous, had a visual acuity of 20/400 or one-twentieth of normal sight. None of the eye specialists he had consulted could give glasses that would help his distance vision or enable him to read. While he had recently retired from business, he had been an avid reader.

In the first lesson, I did not try to get fusion because

of the blindness of the one eye. Relaxation and mobility were emphasized, and at the end of the lesson he was doing letter board No. 5 at approximately five feet.

His homework consisted of lots of sunning, palming, the long swing, mental imagery and counting.

Palming was difficult for him because of an arthritic arm, but he said he would learn to do it with pillows stuffed under his elbows so that there would be no strain.

He came a week later for his second lesson. He had practiced faithfully, exceeding the schedule we had planned. He was able to do board 7 at about seven feet. He was shown how to do alternate sunning and palming and given the domino wheel drill. He promised to start playing solitaire.

On his third lesson he did board 9 at approximately nine feet. We tried fusion with the cord and he was able to get brief glimpses of the V when I put a light on the side of his very bad eye. He also began to read large print in magazine advertisements and said he would also practice this at home. He also said he would go for walks and look far out in the distance.

Several lessons later he told me he had been reading signboards in the distance that he could not see before. We were able to obtain longer periods of fusion with the cord, and he was able to read the letter board at a greater distance.

In the next lesson, we worked with an eye patch on the better eye. With the "dead" eye he read letters about three inches high, white on a black background about a foot away. He was asked to work with a deck of playing cards, picking out one card at a time, while wearing a patch over his better eye, placing the reds in one pile, the blacks in another. He said he would practice this at home.

The following week, he reported that he was enjoying the card drill. He always checked at the end of the sorting by using the other eye to see how many mistakes he had made. He said that his score was improving all the time. At this lesson he did board No. 14 at about thirteen feet with the better eye, and with the weaker eye was able to extend his sight out a little farther on white letters on black backgrounds. He was able to extend the fusion cord farther, too, and was given a black and white ring to use for shifting at home.

His sight continued to improve, and four lessons later he began to see black letters on white backgrounds with the weaker eye at greater distance.

After four more lessons he did over half of letter board No. 1 with the weaker eye at about two feet.

We continued weekly sessions as his distant sight and fusion improved and then started on his close point vision. All told, he had forty-five lessons over a period of two years. His vision in the better eye reached 20/30 and in the weaker eye 20/200, according to his doctor. With both eyes together, he was 20/30. His close point was so good that he read newspapers without glasses.

Donald was a sixteen-year-old boy who, through an eye injury, had developed a cataract. His doctor thought an operation might be advisable, but his father thought they should try vision retraining first. According to his doctor, the sight in the other eye was 20/30 and glasses had been prescribed, although he was told they would not help the sight of the right or cataractous eye. He was given the same type of lessons as Mr. F.

He was a terrific worker. He devoted at least two hours a day, very often three and four hours, to homework. He was diligent in working with a patch. He palmed often in the classroom. After thirty-four lessons he was playing baseball, reading, seemed to have excellent fusion and later, when he went into the armed services, he was given a rating of better than 20/20 in the one eye and 20/20 in the eye that had once had cataract.

Chapter XVIII

Step-by-Step for Other Serious Eye Problems

Of the many other serious eye problems, I have had the experience thus far of applying visual retraining techniques to six—retinitis and chorioretinitis, retinitis pigmentosa, macular degeneration, atrophy of the optic nerve and conical cornea. In every case, diagnosis had been made by a qualified physician and medical care had been given and usually continued to be given. In many cases, there had been frank acknowledgments by doctors that medicine had little, if anything, more to offer to strengthen vision.

Visual retraining techniques brought sight improvement to many—in some, to a surprising degree.

Perhaps part of the reason is that in all sight loss there may be a large element of tension and the techniques help by relieving tension. It's also true that poor habits of seeing are just as common among people with severe disorders as among others. Indeed, in the severely afflicted, as sight begins to diminish and increasingly desperate attempts are made to see, the straining and staring may add to the loss.

Perhaps relaxation and retraining have beneficial effects on the physical ailment itself, helping to improve that. Or it may be that visual retraining only helps by showing how to make the best possible use of the remnants of visual capacity. If sight retraining did nothing more than that, it would, of course, be worthwhile.

The step-by-step program presented here may help you hold your residual sight if you have one of the six serious eye problems mentioned. It may increase your visual acuity. It is not a substitute for medical attention—rather, a helpful adjunct.

RETINITIS AND CHORIORETINITIS

Retinitis, an inflammation of the retina of the eye, is usually associated with an inflammation of the choroid as well. People who have come to me with diagnoses of retinitis or chorioretinitis have usually had a general blurring of vision. In some, central vision had been lost to a marked degree and sight was possible only with side vision. In most, there was an extreme sensitivity to light.

I do not recommend and have never used visual retraining for people who are in the acute stages of retinitis or chorioretinitis, but only after a physician has decided that the acute stage has been terminated.

If you have retinitis or chorioretinitis, the basic twelve-week program presented later in this chapter will be of increased value if you make just a few modifications:

1. Do the sunning for longer periods—if possible, five minutes at a time, eight to ten times a day.
2. Do the palming for six to ten minutes at a time—preferably eight to ten times a day. Mental imagery can be most helpful to you if you concentrate on remembering and imagining fine detail in the center of objects. For example, in visualizing a target, work inward, starting at the outer edges, then visualizing as clearly as possible the bull's-eye itself.
3. If you have lost some side as well as central sight, if there are areas at the periphery of your vision which are somewhat clouded, widening drills are important. The work with the yardstick shifter, Christmas tree lights, red shifter and ring shift will help in clarifying

clouded areas of peripheral vision. Do these drills just a little longer than indicated whenever you can.

The degree of visual impairment produced by retinitis and chorioretinitis varies, of course. Yet, retraining has proved successful in returning useful vision in some severely afflicted cases. One man's vision was so impaired that when he looked straight ahead he saw only a glowing purple ball about three feet in diameter. In order to see anything clearly, he had to turn his whole head to the side so that he was seeing it with peripheral vision. Now he has left only a slight lavender spot of about an inch in diameter. The improvement allows him now to use reading glasses. His distant sight is correspondingly improved; he can now follow the flight of a ball, for example, and catch it successfully.

RETINITIS PIGMENTOSA

Considered to be chronic and progressive in nature, retinitis pigmentosa involves pigmentary degeneration of the retina. It produces night blindness, a progressive loss of sight and contracting field of vision.

If this is your problem, the relaxation drills and those for achieving mobility and centralization and good fusion will be of cardinal importance. You will be helped, too, as you practice accommodation and learn to make maximum use of your mind's functions in good sight.

If you have night blindness, a particular form of mental imagery will help. Spend a good deal of your palming time imagining yourself going from a lighted exterior into a dark interior. For example, imagine that you are descending into a cavern where you see only blackness, with not a glimmer of light anywhere. After you have done this a number of times while palming, you can practice it at other times. And if you close your eyes briefly, think of the blackness of the cavern, then open your eyes and look around, the room in which you are working will appear to be much more brilliantly illuminated.

As you do this little drill, helping yourself to adjust better to darkness, both mentally as well as with the physical eye, your vision outside at night, or in poorly illuminated rooms, will improve.

Changes in light, as well as inadequate light, often bother people with retinitis pigmentosa. They have trouble when going from a strongly lighted place to a dark one or vice versa. If you have the problem, do this in some of your palming: Imagine that you are on a beach and that the sun is very bright, almost blinding. See it that way mentally, and later, when you open your eyes, the light will not seem to be as intense.

You can make use of these techniques, after practice has made them easy, in adjusting to these varying situations in actuality. If you enter a theater and cannot get quickly acclimated to the reduced illumination, close your eyes for just a moment, imagine the cavern, then open your eyes and you'll see better in the darkened theater. Conversely, when you leave a theater or any other poorly illuminated area to go into sunlight, close your eyes for a moment and imagine a sunny beach scene, then open your eyes and you will adjust more rapidly to the increased illumination.

Another good practice is to go into your kitchen at night, leave the door two or three inches ajar so a little crack of light will enter from another room. Stand alongside the kitchen light switch in position so you can see the hot- and cold-water faucets in the sink. With a head motion, look from one faucet to the other five or six times. Flick off the kitchen light and continue to look back and forth from hot- to cold-water faucet. Soon, you will actually see the faucets again in the lesser illumination. Then turn the light back on and look at the faucets again. Repeat the drill three or four more times, turning the light off and on. Practice this at least three or four times a week, and preferably every night.

For an excellent vision-widening drill, put your hands out in front of you, with palms down and thumbs touching. Look directly at the edge of one thumbnail and see if you are aware, at the same time, of the outline of both hands. If you can do this, move the hands a little farther apart and try it again. Continue until you discover the maximum distance at which you can hold them apart and still see outlines of both hands while looking at one thumbnail. Then, with a head motion, look from the little finger tip on one hand to the little finger tip on the other four times. Close your eyes, and with the same head motion, remembering the appearance of the finger tips, mentally look from one to the other. When you open your eyes, you should be able to see the little finger tips more clearly and be able to move your hands another half-inch apart. If you practice this drill for five to ten minutes a day, you will in a few months be able to move your hands many inches farther apart and in the process improve your peripheral vision.

One of my best cases of retinitis pigmentosa was a man who when he started to use these techniques could see an area less than three feet in width at a distance of three feet out in front of him. Today he is regularly playing tennis.

MACULAR DEGENERATION AND ATROPHY OF THE OPTIC NERVE

Macular degeneration, as the term implies, is a degenerative process in the area of keenest vision in the eye, the macular area. Atrophy of the optic nerve involves a degeneration of nerve fibers. In both cases, visual acuity progressively decreases. Sensitivity to light may also be present.

In several dozen cases of atrophy of the optic nerve and macular degeneration the techniques given in the step-by-step procedure at the end of this chapter have brought results ranging from fair to excellent. One woman with macular degeneration for over twenty years had to be led in to see me on her first visit. At a distance of nine inches directly in front of her eyes, she could just barely make out a letter four inches high. She could see a few pale colors but no dark ones. In her last test, at her doctor's office, she saw letters two inches high at a distance of four feet. She can now distinguish dark green, dark blue and is beginning to distinguish red objects. The biggest gain has been in her everyday life. Now she can see the candles in her church, the aisle as she walks to the altar, the lettering on packaged goods such as loaves of bread in the market. She is now able to go many places alone and manage for herself. She has accomplished this after two and one-half years of work. There have been similar good results in some people with atrophy of the optic nerve. Obviously, in such severe conditions, overnight results cannot be expected. Gains are won slowly.

CONICAL CORNEA

This is a non-inflammatory condition in which a conical protrusion of the center of the cornea may cause a high degree of nearsightedness. In some cases, even thick glasses are not enough to help vision and contact lenses may be used.

The techniques in the step-by-step program presented later in this chapter have proved helpful in a number of conical cornea cases. A few modifications increase their value:

1. Much of your palming, and even all of it at the beginning, can be done more effectively while lying down flat on your back.

2. In practicing accommodation, put heavy emphasis on clarity. In your letter board work, for example, if you see the letters clearly at any particular distance, repeat the drill at this distance for four or five days before trying to increase the distance. Aim for greater clarity and greater ease first.

If you have conical cornea but still have relatively good sight, you may be able to disregard the twelve-week program given here, which is intended for the more serious cases, and proceed with the step-by-step techniques used in the chapter on nearsightedness. You can do this if, when you start letter board practice, you can see the larger letters across a card table. In that case, the program in Chapter xi will enable you to make greater and faster progress.

STEP-BY-STEP

In many cases—in fact, in the great majority in my experience—people with serious eye disorders were nearsighted or farsighted even before the retinitis or other major problem developed. If that was true for you, once you complete the program given here, you may be ready to go on, profitably, to do the twelve weeks' work outlined in Chapters xi or xii.

However, if you have had a very great vision loss because of retinitis or one of the other serious problems, you may have to continue the work given in this chapter for six months or even longer before you can bring your vision up to the point where you can begin to tackle your original vision difficulty.

If it's necessary to continue the program given here beyond the twelve-week period, you can repeat it exactly as given or modify it to spend more time on the particular drills which you like best and which seem to be of most value so long as you have a balanced program which includes drills for relaxation, centralization and mobility, fusion and accommodation.

GENERAL HELPS

If your vision is so impaired that you have difficulty in walking because you cannot see far enough ahead, this may be helpful: As you put your left foot forward, look down at the pavement or the floor. Then, as your right foot comes forward, raise your head a little and slide your gaze out a few feet in advance. Look down again as your left foot comes forward, and keep alternating the up and down looks. As you become more proficient in this, you will be able to add a slight sideward head motion, too, which will help you avoid bumping into people on the street.

If there is a great difference in visual acuity between your two eyes, you may reach wide of the mark when you try to pick up or touch objects. If your left eye is weaker, look at the object with both eyes, but move your head quickly three inches to the left and back again, all the time keeping your sight on the object. After a little practice with this, you will be able to touch or pick up anything you want with the first move. If the right eye is weaker, do the reverse. In effect, you are triangulating and in this way determining more accurately where things actually are since, with one eye so markedly weaker than the other, you are unable at this point to get good depth perception. As you build up the sight in your weaker eye and do the fusion work, your depth perception will improve and you will no longer need to triangulate.

BASIC TWELVE-WEEK PROGRAM FOR OTHER SERIOUS EYE PROBLEMS

Every day, every week:

1. Leave your glasses off when doing the drills. Go without them as much as possible at other times—but never to the point of fatigue. Increase your "without glasses" time progressively from week to week.
2. Do the basic relaxation drills (see Chapter III).
   a. Sunning: 4 to 8 sessions of 3-5 minutes each.
   b. Palming with visual imagery: 4 to 8 sessions of 3-5 minutes each.

    c. Long swing: morning and evening, 3 minutes each time.

    d. Short swings: one or more: 2 minutes total.

3. Count objects and colors in free moments (See Chapter IV).

4. Practice vertical shifting (see Chapter IV): whenever possible.

5. Edge objects (see Chapter IV) in free moments: as much as possible.

6. Toss ball (see Chapter IV): 1-3 minutes.

Also each week:

1. See a movie if it does not tire you.

IN ADDITION
Practice each day during the

FIRST WEEK

1. Jumbled numbers (Chap. VI): 1-3 minutes.

2. Reading (Chap. VIII): smallest print you can do with ease, from newspaper headlines to very small print: 5-10 minutes.

3. Letter board (Chap. VI): 5-8 minutes.

4. Cord fusion (Chap. V): 2-4 minutes.

SECOND WEEK

1. Letter board (Chap. VI): a little farther out: 6-8 minutes.

2. Playing card drill (Chap. VI): 5-10 minutes.

3. Solitaire (Chap. IV): 5-10 minutes.

4. Ring shift (Chap. IV): 1-3 minutes.

5. Ruler shift (Chap. IV): 1-3 minutes.

6. Reading (Chap. VIII): newspaper headlines and advertisements: 5-10 minutes.

7. Walking to and from mirror (Chap. xvii): 2 minutes.
8. Cord fusion (Chap. v): 1-3 minutes.

THIRD WEEK

1. Alternate sunning and palming (Chap. iii).
2. Red shifter (Chap. iv): near to far: 1-3 minutes.
3. Jumbled numbers (Chap. vi): 2-4 minutes.
4. Playing card drill (Chap. vi): 5-10 minutes.
5. Reading (Chap. viii): newspaper headlines and magazine advertisements: 5-10 minutes.
6. Walking to and from mirror (Chap. xvii): 2 minutes.
7. Ring fusion or cord fusion (Chap. v): 1-2 minutes, twice a day.

FOURTH WEEK

1. Christmas tree lights (Chap. iv): 2-4 minutes.
2. Letter board (Chap. vi): each eye separately: 10-18 minutes total time.
3. Domino wheels (Chap. vi): both eyes together: 1-3 minutes.
4. Walking to and from mirror (Chap. xvii): 1 minute.
5. Solitaire (Chap. iv): both eyes together: 5-10 minutes.
6. Reading (Chap. viii): newspaper headlines and magazine advertisements, or smaller print: 5-10 minutes.
7. If sight is good enough start on the Gettysburg Address (see p. 111) in smallest print you can see (Chap. viii): 2-4 minutes.
8. Ring fusion (Chap. v): 1-3 minutes.
9. Cord fusion (Chap. v): 1-3 minutes.

FIFTH WEEK

1. Playing card drill (Chap. vi): both eyes together: 5-10 minutes total time.
2. Jumbled numbers (Chap. vi): each eye separately: 3-5 minutes.

3. Domino wheel (Chap. vi): 2-5 minutes.
4. Lights in mirror (Chap. iv): 8-10 minutes.
5. Reading (Chap. viii): newspaper headlines, magazine advertisements or smaller print advertisements: 10-20 minutes.
6. Walking to and from mirror (Chap. xvii): each eye separately: 1 minute; two eyes together: 1-2 minutes.
7. Ring fusion (Chap. v): 1-3 minutes.

SIXTH WEEK

1. Letter board (Chap. vi): each eye separately: 8-15 minutes total time.
2. Playing card drill (Chap. vi): both eyes together: 5-10 minutes.
3. Domino wheel (Chap. vi): 1-2 minutes.
4. Jumbled numbers (Chap. vi): 1-3 minutes.
5. Reading (Chap. viii): newspaper headlines, magazine advertisements or smaller print: 10-20 minutes.
6. Walking to and from mirror (Chap. xvii): each eye separately: 1 minute; both together: 1 minute.
7. Boat fusion (Chap. v): 1-3 minutes.
8. Plate fusion (Chap. v): 1-3 minutes.
9. Cord fusion (Chap. v): 2-3 minutes.

SEVENTH WEEK

1. Domino wheel (Chap. vi): each eye separately: 4-6 minutes total time.
2. Red shifter (Chap. iv): 1 minute.
3. Alternate sunning and palming (Chap. iii): 2 minutes.
4. Playing card drill (Chap. vi): 4-8 minutes.
5. Jumbled letters (Chap. vi): both eyes together: 2-4 minutes.
6. Walking to and from a mirror (Chap. xvii): each eye separately: 1 minute.
7. Reading (Chap. viii): newspaper, magazines and smaller print in this book: 10-25 minutes.

8. Plate fusion (Chap. v): 1-2 minutes.
9. Cord fusion (Chap. v): 2-4 minutes.
10. Ring fusion (Chap. v): 1-3 minutes.

EIGHTH WEEK

1. Playing card drill (Chap. vi): 5-10 minutes.
2. Letter board (Chap. vi): each eye separately: 8-12 minutes total time.
3. Jumbled letters: both eyes together: 3-4 minutes.
4. Solitaire (Chap. x): both eyes together: 5-10 minutes.
5. Ring fusion (Chap. v): 1-3 minutes.
6. Reading (Chap. viii): 10-30 minutes.
7. Walking to and from mirror (Chap. xvii): each eye separately: 1 minute; both eyes together: 1 minute.
8. Ruler fusion (Chap. v): 1-3 minutes.
9. Cord fusion (Chap. v): 1-3 minutes.

NINTH WEEK

1. Red shifter (Chap. iv): 1-3 minutes.
2. Domino wheels (Chap. vi): each eye separately: 4-8 minutes total time.
3. Playing card drill (Chap. vi): 5-10 minutes.
4. Reading (Chap. viii): newspaper headlines or magazine advertisements: 2-4 minutes with each eye.
5. Reading (Chap. viii): small print with both eyes together: 10-30 minutes.
6. Ruler fusion (Chap. v): 1-2 minutes.
7. Cord fusion (Chap. v): 2-3 minutes.

TENTH WEEK

1. Alternate sunning and palming: 1-2 minutes.
2. Solitaire (Chap. iv): each eye separately: 6-10 minutes or more.
3. Letter board (Chap. vi): both eyes together: 4-10 minutes.

4. Jumbled letters (Chap. vi): 1-3 minutes.
5. Reading (Chap. viii): as small print as possible without strain: 10-30 minutes.
6. Walking to and from mirror (Chap. xvii): 1 minute.
7. Ring fusion: 1-3 minutes.
8. Cord fusion (Chap. v): 2-3 minutes.

ELEVENTH WEEK

1. Alternate sunning and palming (Chap. iii): 2 minutes.
2. Lights in mirror (Chap. iv): each eye separately: 2-3 minutes, total 4-6 minutes.
3. Letter board (Chap. vi): each eye separately: 10-18 minutes total time.
4. Domino wheel (Chap. vi): 1-3 minutes.
5. Jumbled letters (Chap. vi): both eyes together: 2-4 minutes.
6. Jumbled numbers (Chap. vi): 2-4 minutes.
7. Reading (Chap. viii): smaller print, if possible without strain: 10-35 minutes.
8. Cord fusion (Chap. v): 2-5 minutes.
9. Plate fusion (Chap. v): 1-4 minutes.
10. Ruler fusion (Chap. v): 1-3 minutes.

TWELFTH WEEK

1. Lights to mirror to letter board to mirror (Chap. xvii): each eye separately: 4-6 minutes.
2. Plate fusion on letter board (Chap. vi): 1 minute.
3. Domino wheel (Chap. vi): 1-3 minutes.
4. Reading (Chap. viii): 10-40 minutes.
5. Solitaire (Chap. iv): 10-15 minutes.
6. Walking to and from mirror (Chap. xvii): 2-4 minutes.
7. Ruler fusion (Chap. v): 1-2 minutes.
8. Cord fusion (Chap. v): 2-3 minutes.
9. See your doctor.

CASE HISTORIES

Retinitis Pigmentosa

Mr. M. S., a man in his early thirties, had retinitis pigmentosa, and, according to his doctor, 20/100 vision in his right eye and 20/200 in his left. He told me that he had night blindness and a very limited field of vision. He could read without glasses but became very tired. He said that his chief problem was one of acute embarrassment as he didn't see immediately things that were handed to him.

The first lesson consisted of basic relaxation and letter board work. He practiced relaxation techniques at home for a week and also did the playing card drill almost every day.

In his second lesson he was able to see slightly smaller size letters a little farther out. I gave him the widening drills. He said, "I'll certainly do these if they can increase my field." I also taught him the drills to help him see better at night.

He began to measure the width of his visual field at a distance of three feet on his red shifter at home. In his fifth lesson he reported that at three feet he thought his field had increased four inches in width. He made an improvement during this lesson and did twelve letters of my letter board 10 at about eleven feet with both eyes.

After he had done part of a smaller board at a shorter distance with the right eye and finished it with both, he got the cord fusion out to about three and a half feet.

I gave him a cord to use at home, and by the following week he could see the V of the cord out another foot and a half.

He came for lessons for almost two years. At the end of that time he was playing tennis, driving a car, and his right eye read better than required when he took his driver's test.

Occasionally when I have met him since his lessons ceased, he has reported that he is seeing well and that he still does sunning, palming and some accommodation and fusion work almost every day.

What has pleased him most is his ability to cope with social situations that had bothered him. And he no longer has difficulty in seeing a proffered hand.

Macular Degeneration

R. S., formerly a secretary, came with a diagnosis of myopia and macular degeneration. She could count fingers at four feet with one eye and at five feet with the other eye. Even with ten-diopter glasses, she had only 20/100 vision. The eye specialist sent me this very complete report regarding her sight.

In her first lesson, we practiced basic relaxation, letter board and cord fusion drills. Occasionally during the cord work, she saw the point of the V at about five feet.

She made up a playing card drill for use at home, but it was a little too difficult for her. In the second lesson I suggested that she play solitaire instead.

After five weeks of solitaire practice, along with fusion, mobility and relaxation work, she was able to do the playing card drill at about three feet. She also could begin to work with the domino wheels.

In a succeeding lesson she was able to work cord fusion consistently at seven to nine feet.

In later lessons she was able to get good ring fusion, and still later succeeded in getting boat and yardstick fusion.

She practiced all the fusion drills faithfully at home and made a big advance in her work with the letter boards.

She spent a good deal of time in the park, counting trees and people and the pigeons that swarmed around. This she called her favorite practice in mobility.

She practiced for a little over a year. Her sight improved greatly. She still wears glasses but now they bring her vision, according to her doctor, close to 20/40 and she is working again as a secretary.

Chorioretinitis

C. W., an accountant, had had a series of hemorrhages some years before, and medical examination indicated a number of exudates. Because of his poor vision, he had not been able to work at his profession for four years. Glasses, he said, did not help at all.

In his first lesson he was shown the basic relaxation drills. Then we tried a large letter board and fusion on the cord. The letters were not clear as his only vision was side vision, but he did get glimpses of the fusion cord V at about five feet. He was asked to toss a ball as part of his home practice and also to play solitaire and was given a ring for shifting and asked to use it several times a day. He practiced faithfully, and, in his second lesson, he did all of a letter board, a slightly smaller size and a little farther away than in the first lesson. He also saw the letters a little more directly in front of him.

After a few weeks, he was able to do the playing card drill at home. In his home practice, he began to stretch the fusion cord out five or six feet farther. Then he mastered ring fusion and boat fusion. These techniques, plus use of the red shifter and ruler shifting, helped him to begin to read newspaper headlines and the large print in magazine advertisements.

His distant sight kept improving, and he began to play catch instead of just tossing a ball.

After almost a year of lessons he returned to his doctor who told him that his exudates were gone.

He continues his practice and now is able to work at his profession with glasses on.

Conical Cornea

L. W., a young woman with a doctor's diagnosis of conical cornea and 20/400 vision in each eye, had worn glasses for years, including contact lenses.

In the first lesson she was given the basic relaxation work and did one large letter board.

She could read fine print very close to her, and so was given the two domino wheels for near to far work. I also asked her to make up the playing card drill.

The next week she reported that she was now doing the playing card drill eight inches farther out than the first time she had done it at home. She also said that she could do the domino wheels two inches farther out than when she started.

In succeeding lessons, she progressively read smaller letter boards farther out. She reported similar improvement in her home fusion practice. She was ingenious in finding extra practice work such as watching flashing signs at night.

Several lessons later, I gave her an eye patch for use at home in the recommended drills.

She went to one movie each week and said that she had moved back from the first to the eighth row. She remarked that, although the screen was blurred at the latter distance, it was no more so than when she had had to sit in the first row.

At the end of six months, her doctor prescribed weaker lenses. She continued her lessons and her practice work at home until she reached what her doctor said was 20/70 vision. She does almost everything except drive a car without glasses. In fact, she has a much weaker pair than her original ones for driving and no longer wears contact lenses.

Atrophy of Optic Nerve

Mrs. L. T. came to my office with a doctor's diagnosis of atrophy of the optic nerve, 20/400 vision and limited field. She had worn reading glasses for twelve years, then bifocals for another twelve.

After basic relaxation work in the first lesson, she did one-half of the largest letter board at six feet.

Because she had a diagnosis of high blood pressure, she

was not given the long swing. The light for sunning was placed three feet farther out than usual because she said it bothered her when it was closer.

Her homework consisted of the basic relaxation techniques, counting, solitaire, red shifter and cord fusion drills.

In her second lesson she did the next smaller letter board about eight inches farther out. She also extended the cord out another foot.

I asked her to make a playing card drill to use at home and gave her a ring for shifting.

Her improvement after this lesson was more rapid as she doubled the time spent in sunning and palming. Up until this time she had done the two rather sketchily.

She did the playing card drill five days a week, and worked the red shifter and ring shift twice each a day.

In the following lessons she was taught to do alternate sunning and palming. She reported that light was not bothering her as much as it had before and that she thought her field was a little wider. At this lesson she saw some words in magazine advertisements and newspaper headlines.

During her next lesson she did a smaller letter board and gained two more feet on cord fusion. She got glimpses of ring fusion also.

I asked her to toss a ball at home.

Her improvement continued. She had two more weeks of lessons before she had to move across the country. At that point, the doctor reported her sight was 20/100. He also told her that her field had improved. She could read newspaper headlines down to half-inch size easily.

Chapter XIX

Step-by-Step for the Blind

Can *blind* people be helped to gain back sight by techniques of visual re-education? The answer is—yes, in some cases. For a number have regained useful vision.

There are, of course, various degrees of blindness. The totally blind person does not even see light. His eyes see no difference between day or night, between a dark or brightly lighted room.

There are blind people who have light perception. While they can make out no objects, they are aware of light. They can tell the difference between day and night, and sense where the windows are in a room.

There are also the blind who have at least slight object perception. They can, for example, notice that there are pictures on a wall even if they are unable to tell what they are.

Whatever your degree of blindness, if someone is reading this book to you and will work with you to see that you are doing the techniques correctly, you will enjoy trying to improve your sight. Perhaps you will be one of those who will benefit. There can be no guarantee of success. But if you are willing to devote some time each day for a trial period of six or eight weeks, you should within that time be able to tell whether it will be worthwhile to continue. For even if you are totally blind, within that time, if the techniques will help you at all, they will have brought some light perception.

Whatever your degree of blindness now, in fact, you can try the techniques for two months. If, at the end of that time, you're not certain that you're benefiting—if you think you may be but then again think that perhaps you're only imagining improvement—continue for another month, and by that time you will have no doubts. There will be more definite improvement—or none.

The trial is worthwhile. For there is not much effort involved.

GAINING LIGHT PERCEPTION

If you are totally blind, your first efforts will be directed toward trying to achieve light perception.

The techniques for this are few and simple. You should sun and palm, exactly as described in Chapter III, eight times a day, spending five minutes for each session.

While you're palming, use mental imagery. Try to imagine that you are actually seeing again. Remember back to when you could really see, and then in your mind's eye, try to picture as many objects as possible, especially those you remember with pleasure. This may take a little effort at first, but persist and the imagery will become easier for you. Go on to visualize numbers and the letters of the alphabet.

Do the lazy-daisy head motion drill, as described in Chapter III. If it seems a little strange to begin with, you'll probably soon find it pleasant and relaxing. Do it at least three or four times a day—for a minute or two each time. And if you enjoy doing it more often, all to the good.

These are your beginning techniques. After two or three weeks of them, have someone swing the light you use for sunning toward your closed eyes and then away again. Indicate when you sense the light on your closed lids and when it has been moved away. Are you right? Are you beginning to be able to sense it at least some of the time?

When you can always tell, when you can also see windows and lights with your eyes open, you will have the light perception you need to continue on with other techniques designed to help you progress toward object perception.

GAINING OBJECT PERCEPTION

If you have light perception to begin with, or achieve it by the techniques just described, you can work with the following techniques for helping to bring object perception.

Do the sunning and palming six to ten times a day, about five to eight minutes at a time. Do the mental imagery while palming, remembering how things looked when you did have sight, picturing them and numbers and the letters of the alphabet, in particular.

Do the lazy-daisy head swing for relaxation several times a day.

If you have a rocking chair, rock in it at least some of the time each day and, while rocking, imagine that you are seeing objects across the room. In effect, this is mental imagery with your eyes open. The rocking motion will help you relax and it also serves to break any stare for it's difficult to stare as you move.

Take an orange or a rubber ball and pass it from one hand to the other, following it with a head motion—just imagining you see it. Do this two to three times a day for three or four minutes at a time.

Perhaps your hand was the last thing you saw. Pass your hand back and forth close to and in front of your eyes three or four times.

Follow it with a head motion and *imagine* that you are seeing it. It will probably be the first thing you actually do see again. But for now, just imagine. Do this little drill as often as possible each day.

Use a string of Christmas tree lights for shifting and mobility. Place them where you can see them—perhaps

only two feet away to start. Gradually, you should be able
to see them a little farther out. Do not strain in your endeavor
to see them at greater and greater distances. It is better to
see them with increasing clarity close to you. At first you
may see only the white and the yellow lights. Then when
you can see the red your sight should be better. The green
light is next in difficulty, and the blue is the most difficult of
all. Don't stare at the lights. With a head motion, begin
with the one at the left and sweep your gaze across the
lights to the last one at the other end, then back again. Do
this for two or three minutes at a time. Do it three to five
times a day.

And these are all the techniques you will use in trying to
advance from light perception to object perception. They
may seem simple. They are, indeed. Yet they have proved
effective.

If they are going to be helpful for you, when can you
expect results? There can be no precise answer. It may take
only a month or two. It is much more likely to require
three or four months. But you will be able to tell, within a
month, whether you are going to benefit. By that time, you
should begin to notice just a little improvement at least. And
if you do, you can continue to work with the expectation that
as the weeks go by you will make further progress.

When you do achieve object perception—that is, when
you can see your hands and fingers and make out, even
dimly, the furniture in a room and the frames of pictures on
the wall, you are ready to begin the twelve weeks' work outlined below for those with object perception.

ACHIEVING USEFUL VISION

If you have object perception to begin with, or have
achieved it with the techniques already described, you are
ready for a more advanced program which is designed to
help you improve your vision to the point where you can see

large letters on a board held across a card table from you—
a distance of about two and a half feet. And, at that point,
there will be other work which you can do to improve your
vision still further.

The work you are to do for the next twelve weeks is outlined below. In most cases, the techniques are exactly like
those described in the beginning chapters of this book.

These additional comments and suggestions may be helpful.

Understandably enough, many blind people have forgotten how to look and have lost all curiosity. They tap their
cane on the sidewalk but never look down at the place they
are tapping. You must look around with a head motion even
if you do not see much.

Some blind people wear glasses even though they say they
see no better with them on. If you use glasses, take them off
whenever you're doing any of the drills.

All of the relaxation work is essential. Sun and palm at
least as much as called for—more, if you can. Do the mental
imagery when you palm. Have someone read over for you
what has been said earlier in this chapter about imagery and
also the longer discussion of it in Chapter III.

Don't try the long swing unless you are very sure on your
feet. Even then your assistant should hold onto you. Later
you may be able to do it alone by placing two straight chairs
with their backs facing your hips and holding a hand on the
back of each chair. If your assistant can't always be with
you for this technique, you can swing your shoulders and
your head from side to side as you sit in a chair.

A rocking chair is a wonderful aid, but if you don't have
one you can sit in a straight chair and rock up and down
with your body. Let your head go with your body and let
your gaze go with your head. This will help achieve relaxation and increase mobility, too.

When you toss or juggle your ball or orange, follow it with your nose.

Counting objects and colors, especially colors, will be difficult for you, but you can practice in short sessions. As soon as possible begin counting colors in magazine advertisements.

Get some black cardboard. An art supply shop will usually have it. Have someone cut it up for you into four-inch squares and draw, with white poster paint, the capital letters of the alphabet three inches high, one to a square.

Mix up these letter cards on a table in front of you. Then pick up one letter at a time, glance at it briefly, call it and lay it down. Don't stare. Make your look a very quick one. If someone can be present to check your work, good. But if not, practice anyhow. And no matter whether you do well or not, whether you call each letter perfectly, you'll improve as you go along. But you'll improve only if you use correct vision habits—if, instead of staring and studying, you use quick glances and blink fairly frequently, every five to ten seconds.

Later, as your sight improves, you can progress to work with two-inch-high letters and then to one-inch letters.

If your assistant has the time, you can practice by calling the letters as he stands in front of you and holds them up one at a time. Gradually, he can move backward to increase the distance.

Later, too, as your sight improves you can practice arranging the letters into words on the table in front of you.

In doing the sorting work with playing cards, you may have to start with special jumbo-size cards, then later use regular-size cards.

Do not work too hard. In the twelve-week program, no time limits are given except for sunning and palming. Be your own judge of how long you can work without fatigue. Stop often, even right in the middle of a drill, and sun and palm.

By the end of the twelfth week, your sight may have improved enough so you are ready to try to increase it still more with the program to be found in the step-by-step chapter devoted to the problem that may have caused your original sight loss—glaucoma or cataracts, for example.

You will be ready for such further work when you're able to distinguish one-inch-high letters across a card table. If you are still not up to this after the twelve weeks of work given here, keep on until you are. Do not be discouraged. If you see the slightest improvement in your vision, keep working.

Believe that you can see. Make each day an adventure, a voyage of discovery in the world around you, a re-exploration of a world of form, of shape, of color, of beauty which you had forgotten but which you want to see again.

BASIC TWELVE-WEEK PROGRAM FOR THOSE WITH OBJECT PERCEPTION

Every day, every week:

1. Leave your glasses off when doing the drills. Go without them as much as you can at other times—but never to the point of fatigue. Increase your "without glasses" time progressively from week to week.
2. Do the basic relaxation drills (see Chapter III).
   a. Sunning: 8 times a day, 5 minutes at a time.
   b. Palming with visual imagery: 8 times a day, 5 minutes at a time.
   c. Long swing: twice a day.
   d. Lazy-daisy and cogwheel swings, 8 times a day: 8-16 minutes total time.
3. Count objects and colors (see Chapter IV) in free moments.
4. Practice vertical shifting (see Chapter IV): whenever possible.

5. Rock in a rocking chair.
6. Toss ball or orange.

IN ADDITION
Practice each day during the

FIRST WEEK

Nothing more.

SECOND WEEK

1. Large 3-inch letters (Chap. xix). Go through alphabet if possible. Close and remember letters often.
2. Christmas tree lights (Chap. xix).

THIRD WEEK

1. Large 3-inch letters, through alphabet (Chap. xix).
2. Christmas tree lights (Chap. xix).

FOURTH WEEK

1. Large 3-inch letters, twice through alphabet (Chap. xix).
2. Sort deck of cards into two piles, black cards and red cards.

FIFTH WEEK

1. If you have some sight in each eye, try 3-inch letters with one eye and then with the other, using an eye patch (Chap. xix).
2. Sort cards (if possible sort according to suits). Otherwise continue to sort according to red and black.
3. Large red shifter (Chap. iv).
4. Count colors in magazine ads.

SIXTH WEEK

1. Try 2-inch letters. If too small, return to 3-inch size (Chap. xix).

2. Sort deck of cards twice.
3. Christmas tree lights (Chap. XIX).
4. Large red shifter (Chap. IV).
5. Count colors in magazine ads.

SEVENTH WEEK

1. Through alphabet twice with 2-inch letters if possible, otherwise with 3-inch letters.
2. Try game of solitaire. If too difficult, sort deck.
3. Christmas tree lights in mirror (Chap. IV).
4. Ring shift (Chap. IV).

EIGHTH WEEK

1. Sort letters with each eye if possible.
2. Solitaire or sort playing cards.
3. Ring shift (Chap. IV).
4. Red shifter (Chap. IV).
5. Count colors in magazine ads.

NINTH WEEK

1. Try large-size letters in graduated print (Chap. VIII). If too difficult, return to letters used before.
2. Solitaire.
3. Domino wheel (Chap. VI).
4. Ruler shift (Chap. IV).
5. Try cord fusion (Chap. V) if you have some sight in each eye.

TENTH WEEK

1. Christmas tree lights in mirror, each eye separately and then both eyes together (Chap. IV).
2. Letter cards, through alphabet two or three times.
3. Domino wheel (Chap. VI).
4. Count colors in magazine ads.
5. Cord fusion (Chap. V).

ELEVENTH WEEK

1. Sort letter cards, each eye separately and both eyes together.
2. Make words from letters on table in front of you.
3. Ring shift (Chap. IV).
4. Ruler shift (Chap. IV).
5. Cord fusion (Chap. V).

TWELFTH WEEK

1. Christmas tree lights in mirror: each eye and both eyes together (Chap. IV).
2. Domino wheel (Chap. VI).
3. Words on table.
4. Ring shift (Chap. IV).
5. Cord fusion (Chap. V).

CASE HISTORY

Two days after a brain operation Mr. D. L. had suddenly lost sight. His right eye had only light perception. With his left eye he could see letters about three inches high when he held them close to the eye.

In his sighted days he had been an important business executive and had a very good mind. When I said, "I don't know how much we can improve your sight," he said, "What have I got to lose?"

In the first lesson, he was taught basic relaxation. He was also asked to get a ball and move it from one hand into the other, watching it just as if he saw it perfectly.

I asked him to practice for two weeks concentrating on mental imagery, too, then return.

In his second lesson he was able to see letters at a distance of three feet. He called all the letters in the alphabet, making only an occasional error which he corrected immediately. I gave him a large red shifter and asked him to use it several times a day. I suggested a good deal of rocking, too.

When he went for an automobile ride, he practiced mental imagery, imagining that he could see the dials on the dashboard, the road in the distance, a white house to the left, a red barn to the right, etc.

In his fourth lesson I had asked him to sort playing cards according to red or black, and when he came back for his next lesson he announced, "Sorting according to red or black is too easy. I sort them according to suits and my wife checks them. I make very few mistakes."

He was making steady progress in reading letters, each time a little farther out, and in the sixth lesson I gave him an eye patch and asked him to move his hand slowly back and forth in front of his right eye. He was able to see his hand. I gave him the patch and asked him to practice at home.

In his next lesson he was able to distinguish four letters, about three inches high, white letters on a black background, with the right eye.

During this lesson he showed such improvement of sight that I consulted a surgeon regarding his case. I felt that it would be unfair to have him make only a temporary improvement of sight. The surgeon said, "Keep on, you're on the right track. Any improvement that you can get will hold."

After I relayed the surgeon's statement, he had a further magnificent gain.

I started tossing a large ball to him from only a few feet away. I told him I was an expert ball player and the ball would always come into his expectant hands. Thus he had no fear of being hurt.

I increased the distance in successive lessons up to ten feet. Then he said, "You can just toss it, I'm not afraid of it any more."

A few weeks later he told me that he was doing a near to far drill from the red shifter in his hand to a picket fence twenty yards away.

He now came to his lessons without a guide.

He said in a later lesson that while he palmed he often visualized himself playing nine holes of golf.

He is now in business again, plays golf and enjoys a normal life.

I still have a letter he wrote while on a business trip. In it he said: "This is the first letter I myself have written in two and a half years. I felt it should be to you."

Chapter XX

Help for the Child:
A Guide for Parents

Overcoming the handicap of defective vision, important at any age, is especially rewarding for a child. For better vision can play an important role throughout his lifetime—in personality and social development, in schoolwork and, later, in his whole career.

For children the techniques presented in earlier chapters, the step-by-step programs, too, have proved to be as effective as for adults. If your child has poor vision, a trained teacher, especially one experienced in working with youngsters, can speed and ease the process of improvement. She's trained not only to use techniques skillfully but to understand his visual handicaps, his need for praise and the emotional problems of a child who competes with normal-sighted children. Yet, if one is not available, and if you are willing to give time and thought to the project, you can do much, and perhaps all that is needed to help your child.

The few modifications and variations in techniques and the suggestions for working with a child which are presented in this chapter should prove of value. They are based on my own experience and that of many of my teachers. They are designed to simplify visual retraining, to make it more appealing to, and practical for, children—even those of preschool age.

If your child has good vision now, you can help him to maintain it. Preventing sight loss, especially during periods that may be critical for his vision and, beyond that, helping him to firmly establish sound habits of using his sight which will stand him in good stead all his life, are worthwhile goals—and fortunately can be achieved with comparatively little effort on your part or his.

OVERCOMING DEFECTIVE VISION

1. THE WILL TO SEE BETTER

Not long ago, an eleven-year-old girl was brought to my office by her concerned mother. The child was nearsighted and wore glasses all the time. To one of my first questions— did she like wearing them, would she mind having to go on wearing them—her reply was a flip, "Sure, why not?"

Her mother broke in quickly to explain, "That's my fault. When glasses were first prescribed for her myopia, she hated them, but I kept telling her over and over again that she looked prettier when she wore them."

It took eight months before the mother, following my suggestion to wait, was able to phone me and announce excitedly, "She's ready to start lessons now. Yesterday and again this morning she refused to wear her glasses." Lessons were started then. After only twelve of them, she read 20/20 for the school nurse.

It would have been a waste of time to have begun the lessons earlier. If there is no real interest in improving vision, the job of trying to help bring it about is extremely difficult, if not impossible. Fully as much as the adult, the child must have a compelling desire, a thorough motivation, to see better.

If your child has it, you're ready to start helping him. If not, how can you get him to actively want better vision?

In my experience, commands are of little value.

If your boy wants to grow up to be a pilot, you can explain that pilots generally must have excellent vision. If he wants to be an athlete, you can point out that few athletes wear glasses.

Working on the vanity of a girl may help. You might underline the fact that few movie stars or TV actresses wear glasses at work. You might encourage her to draw the conclusion that most people are better looking without glasses.

It may take months of indirect persuasion, of artful implantation of an appreciation of the importance of good vision before your child is eager to work for it. But the time and effort will be well spent, and improvement will be the more certain after that.

2. PARENTAL ATTITUDE

Your own attitude, as the parent, will be an important factor in your child's progress.

You will need to be patient and understanding. Overnight results aren't to be expected. It's important not only that you avoid making excessive demands of the child, but that you try to make the whole process of improvement more a matter of fun than a harsh chore.

It's often true that one parent can work better with a child than the other. Do a little experimenting to find out which one it is in your family. In any case, it will help to make the child appreciate more deeply the importance of improvement in sight if both parents take an active interest.

From the beginning, compliment the child for each step forward—no matter how small. Praise is a vital stimulant. It buoys up adults. It's even more powerful for children.

3. MODIFICATIONS AND VARIATIONS

If your child is nearsighted, the program in Chapter XI should be followed. The farsighted child should do the work presented in Chapter XII. Similarly, if another problem is involved, the program for that particular problem presented in an earlier chapter should be used. And these suggestions should prove helpful:

a. Sunning and Palming

It is usually more effective for a child to have a regular routine for sunning and palming than to practice them at odd moments. Before or after breakfast, after the midafternoon snack, after dinner, between television shows and just before retiring are all good times. If your child likes some better than others, you can let him decide which times to drop as a concession to keeping the others.

If the child finds sunning and palming tedious, especially in the beginning, be firm without making him hate the techniques. Offer rewards if you like—perhaps a movie or an extra few minutes of TV. Best of all, stay with him during the practice. If he's very young, he'll probably like to have you read or tell him a story while he suns. Stories are especially good during palming; you can use them then to help him achieve mental imagery.

b. Mobility and Centralization

Children generally like the drills with the tree lights. Those using dice, ball and cards are often favorites. And, since any game that involves motion is good for mobility practice, you can supplement or vary the drills described in Chapter IV with many others that children will enjoy—for example, rolling a ball or tossing a bean bag.

Many children seem to be particularly enchanted by speed, and if your child balks at just counting colors and objects, try making a game of counting them within a time limit. You can also make a game of tossing a few pebbles or coins into the air and having the child count them as they come down.

To get a child started on vertical and horizontal shifting,

it's often helpful to call attention to objects or colors in various places. Do not ask, "Can you see that tennis ball?" Say, rather, "See that tennis ball go back and forth."

Most children like the long and short swings if they can do them to music—and this is all to the good.

c. Fusion

In my experience, the average child likes the fusion techniques if he does not have to do them for more than a few minutes at a time. Brief sessions, several times a day, will usually prove better than one long session. Color, too, is helpful in fusion work. One of my teachers reported that a child who did not like cord fusion became quite fond of it after she (the child) got the idea of using a number of cords of various colors. Chapter xv contains other suggestions for use of color in fusion which can be adapted for your child's program.

d. Accommodation

For the very young, boards made up of animals cut from a book can be substituted for letter boards. Or, for a child who cannot read, copying letters is good practice. Instead of looking from letters in his hands to those in the distance and calling the latter, he can look at the distant letters on the board, then print them in the same order on a piece of paper.

You can also substitute lotto games for the letter boards. There are various types with pictures of flowers and other objects. The large board with rows of pictures can be placed at a distance and the small pictures matched to it.

Many boys collect picture cards of planes, baseball players, boxers, etc. A double set of these can also be used for accommodation practice. Paste one set on a piece of cardboard for use at the distance and the other set can be used for matching.

e. Toys and Games

You can help improve your child's vision by selecting toys which have vision retraining as well as play value. Any toy that revolves, jumps, rolls or otherwise has motion—a spinning top, flying plane, mechanical boat, car or train, for example—is good for mobility.

Games and sports can also be helpful. Jigsaw puzzles, checkers, chess and others that involve a great deal of staring should be avoided. But there are many that are excellent because they involve motion and require changing focus for near and far. Among them: Ping-pong, tennis, baseball, basketball, bowling, skating, archery, hockey, pitching horseshoes.

f. Blackboard Practice

If your child has difficulty in reading the blackboard in school, you can help by working with a small blackboard at home. Explain that seeing is done by means of comparison and contrast. Demonstrate that on a blackboard, there is contrast between the white of the chalk and the black of the board. Call his attention to differences in the height of letters—for example, the shortness of the longhand a, the tallness of the l, the low g that dips below other letters.

For practice, write on the blackboard a list of wild animals. Tell the child what the list includes—tiger, giraffe, bear, etc. Then, while he's seated or standing at a distance where the writing is slightly blurred, have him try to make out the letters coming above, below and on the line. Ask him to guess which animal it is.

Ask him to close his eyes, too, to try to see, behind his closed lids, a deep blackness like the very darkest night. Then have him open his eyes, and the white chalk on the board will appear just a bit whiter against the black background.

Next, write a list of games—football, baseball, tennis, hockey, etc.—and have him try to read this from a foot farther back. He will probably be able to do it with no more difficulty than he read the first group.

The gain of a whole foot won't hold to the next session—perhaps only a few inches will. But continued practice—several times a week for a period of five to fifteen minutes each time—will help him build distant vision. Each time he gains a little extra distance, even though vision is blurred at that distance, he will gain a little more clarity at the previous distance.

You will find a fuller discussion of blackboard practice in the next chapter which may be helpful.

g. Conference with Teacher

If your child has an understanding, co-operative teacher, a conference with her will be worthwhile.

She may be willing to seat him near enough to the blackboard so he can see without strain—and possibly without glasses. She may also allow him to look out the window from time to time to stretch his sight and permit him to palm occasionally.

These concessions may seem small yet will be most helpful in reinforcing your efforts to improve the child's sight.

Possibly she will be willing and able to go further and adopt some of the suggestions in Chapter xxi for the benefit of your child and the whole class.

PREVENTING POOR SIGHT

As a parent, you can play an important role in helping to prevent sight loss in your child.

Often the beginning of vision difficulty is heralded by blinkless staring and by trick vision—peering up or down unnaturally, or out of the corners of the eyes, or half closing the eyes to see. Such habits are to be discouraged—if possible, in the bud stage. The earlier they're detected, the easier they are to root out.

A particularly critical period for sight comes with the school years. If the child has been a healthy preschool youngster, he has been in and out of doors all day long, his activities have been varied, he has used his sight for distance as well as close point. Now a good portion of his time is being spent in the classroom. His use of distance sight is limited. He is being asked to concentrate his attention. He may be subject to mental strain—and to emotional strain as well.

A good starting point is to check his homework habits. Correct him if he hunches over his work, straining to concentrate and to get through it. Give him comfortable working space and encourage him to work in relaxed fashion, to look up now and then, changing focus, even to get up and move around occasionally.

Check, too, to see that his reading is done properly— that he holds the book at normal reading distance and slightly below eye level. There should be good light for the reading—not only on the reading material itself but in the rest of the room so that he can look up from the book now and then to change focus and see objects about the room.

As a parent, you can and should exercise some supervision over how your child views television. By applying the principles discussed in Chapter x, you can help to prevent harm to the child's vision and, more positively, make TV viewing a helpful factor in the establishment of good visual habits.

You may be able to aid your child's vision, too, by helping him to like his teacher and his schoolwork if he does not already do so. As pointed out earlier, there seems to be a definite correlation between emotions and sight. Many of my sight students have traced the beginning of their visual problem to a time in their life when they were exposed to a teacher they disliked or a subject they loathed.

If your child dislikes his teacher, it may help if you invite her to dinner or to a Saturday luncheon. Once she has been in your home, the chances are that she will seem a little less strange and a little more human to the child and that he will like her better. It's also possible that she may subsequently show him little extra attentions that will help change his dislike to liking.

If your child dislikes a particular subject, you may be able to help by working with him at home. Your efforts need not be in the direction of trying to reinforce the teaching he receives in school. Rather, you can try to develop his interest in the subject. I taught history for several years, and many boys who hated it at first began to like it after I suggested, for outside reading, adventure books with historical backgrounds. If history as taught in the classroom seems remote, entirely academic, completely uninteresting, such outside reading may help to show it in its true light and build the child's interest. If mathematics is his pet hate, perhaps you can set him to playing games in which mathematics is used. Anything you can do to help your child like his schoolwork will be of great importance in preventing emotional strain and its consequences to the sight

Not least of all, you can actively teach your child the principles of good sight—and encourage him to practice some of the techniques for applying them.

He will not need to follow any detailed program of work such as is necessary for the child with a sight loss. Instead, he can use a few techniques each day—during the day—in casual rather than formal practice.

Teach him to shift from near to far and far to near all during the day, to count and edge occasionally, to use a short swing when he feels tired or tense. Encourage him to do a few minutes of the long swing after completing his homework and just before retiring, in order to relax his eyes and his whole body for a good night's sleep. See Chapters IX and x for many other suggestions that are as helpful in keeping good sight as in retrieving it.

One of the most important assets you can endow your child with is an understanding of how to develop and maintain the good visual habits that will help to keep his sight perfect throughout his life.

Chapter XXI

Help for the Child:
A Guide for Teachers

Six and a half million grade-school children in the United States today need but are not receiving eye care. This is the disheartening conclusion reached in a pioneering study made by the National Society for the Prevention of Blindness in collaboration with The Children's Bureau. If these children are like those discovered in another recent survey in the public schools of St. Louis, Missouri, only 25 per cent of them ever complain about their handicap; the rest just suffer in silence.

Vision difficulty can affect a child in many ways. Poor posture, inferior manual skills and personality disturbances are often linked with it. Specialists of the Dyslexia Institute at Northwestern University estimate that fully 70 per cent of school failures are the result of reading difficulties which, very often, trace back to poor sight.

The problem of inadequate vision in our children is enormous. But I believe that it is far from hopeless, that much can be done in our schools—with little effort and at virtually no cost—to help rebuild sight in many children and preserve and strengthen it in all.

"Bright spring sunshine floods the first grade room at Holy Rosary School these spring days, but you don't see fretting youngsters shielding their eyes or asking to have the curtains lowered.

"In the second grade not a child has appeared at school with new glasses this year, although normally at least one or two of the class by now would need glasses.

"Upstairs, high school girls are learning to use their eyes 'sensibly,' and among the Dominican nuns, who staff the faculty, some have abandoned glasses after wearing them for many years."

Thus begins a news account in the Seattle *Post-Intelligencer* of April 16, 1950, which goes on to relate that this is "all part of the 'eye training' being carried on in several Seattle parochial schools under direction of nuns who were trained in the specialty at Seattle University by Clara Hackett."

In the article, too, there appears this statement: "Results so far indicate that the lessening of eye strain has a definite, generally good effect on the work and behavior of the children throughout the day."

The "eye training" program used could hardly be more simple. From their first day in school, up to the time they're ready for college, the children are taught and given daily opportunities to practice the basic relaxation techniques of sunning, palming and swinging.

It takes little time and no equipment to have a class of children take a few breaks on a sunny day and stand facing the windows, letting the sun shine on their closed lids. And on any day there are many opportunities for brief periods of palming and long swings.

There come moments, anyhow, in any classroom when minds wander and children become restless, when the wise teacher calls a halt for a seventh-inning stretch, a brief respite before going on with classwork. Sunning, palming and swinging, used in such moments, provide a release from tension and at the same time help vision.

These three drills alone make up the whole formal program used to help protect and strengthen the eyesight of children in the Seattle parochial schools.

Such a program is universally applicable. As a teacher, you might like to work for its adoption in your school system. Perhaps, in the meantime, it might be feasible for you to put it into immediate use in your own classroom.

With an understanding of the few essentials of good vision, there is much else that you can do—and will find practical to do—to correct poor habits of seeing and help to establish proper ones among your students.

Accommodation is one of the essentials. Our eyes were designed for seeing near and far—and should be used according to the design. They may be abused when, much of the time and for long periods at a time, they're glued to the near point. An attitude of defeatism has grown up around the "fact" that in our civilization, beginning in our schools, little opportunity exists for eye accommodation and that failing eyesight may be a penalty we inevitably have to pay for our modern way of living.

But I do not think this is an established "fact" at all. Much of our work and living, it's true, is close work and indoor living. But the opportunity for accommodation, for proper use of the eyesight, remains. We can demonstrate it in our classrooms, and, once aware of it, our students can find it outside the classroom.

As a child I was exposed to many teachers—and later, as a schoolteacher myself, I found many among my colleagues—who, with the best will, insisted on imposing a discipline: "Pay attention. Keep your eyes on your work. Don't look up from that book." This is supposed to be good for the mind, although there is very grave doubt that it is. In any case, it is ruinous for the sight.

The teacher wise to the needs of a child's vision will permit him to do what he seems to do by instinct—look up and away, now and then, from the printed page to shift his focus. She will even interrupt reading assignments at intervals to have children look at a map or some other object in the room in order to shift focus, and she will allow and encourage them to look out the window from time to time and certainly at the end of a reading assignment.

The habit of looking up and away from print at frequent intervals is one that should be firmly established in the classroom. And students should be taught to do the same thing in all their close work—both in and out of the classroom.

Other good reading habits can be taught, too—and they involve more than reading with good posture and good lighting.

Recently, in an article addressed to educators, a grade-school teacher who had studied with me to help rebuild her own sight wrote: "Instructors have done some terrible things to pupils' vision by insisting that they *spread* their vision, comprehend an entire sentence at a glance. Still others try to make for fast reading by teaching the pupil to glance wide and strenuously at a whole page. Teach yourselves and the children to become 'machine-gun' readers instead. We want our eyes to read single words, one at a time, with the steadiness and rapidity of machine-gun fire. 'Shotgun' readers are slow readers, with the added handicap of eventual vision loss. Boys take to this simile readily. They realize that a shotgun fires many scattered shots into the air at once. The bullets spread but few get near the target."

I heartily endorse her plea. We see best with the central, most sensitive portion of the retina, as noted many times earlier in this book. Mobility and centralization are essential for good vision. Shotgun reading tends to immobilize the sight and prevent centralization.

In your classroom, in other work as well as reading, you can in many simple ways help children to make their sight more mobile and centralized.

When a child writes, teach him to watch the point of his pen or pencil, shifting his gaze to follow it instead of staring at the paper.

If a child looks up and stares as he tries to think of a word, teach him to close his eyes while searching his mind so that he will not be staring.

Children often begin to strain their vision when they make an effort to take in something unfamiliar. They may stare unblinkingly at a new word on the blackboard as if trying to gobble it up. It's helpful in overcoming this to have a large wall calendar at the front of the classroom and to encourage children to shift their gaze from time to time from the blackboard to the calendar. The shifting, in place of staring, will help to relax the sight. It seems also to relax the mind. Frequently, when the child shifts back again to the unfamiliar, he is more likely to be able to comprehend it.

Teach your pupils, too, that one of the best ways to rest the sight is to use it purposefully rather than to stare vacantly at any time. Picking out the most minute details of the material in a window drape is far more restful than simply staring at the over-all drape.

Squinting, cocking the head to one side, peering over the tops of the eyes with lowered head, reading or gazing through a rolled sheet of paper held to one eye—these are all forms of trick vision.

You'll help children's sight a great deal if you're alert for and correct these habits.

Many children experience their first visual difficulty with blackboard work.

Inadequate lighting of the board may be one reason. If schools used light brackets extending out from the top and throwing the light back on the board, I believe there would be much less failure in the vision of school children.

Many schools have begun to use green boards which have some sight-saving value because they provide greater contrast. Even as they become lighter during the day's use, it is easier to pick out the white of the chalk against light green than against the dull gray that an ordinary blackboard soon becomes.

Yet blackboards can be kept blacker for greater contrast and easier seeing. Children like to do classroom chores. Let them take turns keeping the boards clean and black. It will help, too, if you bear down on the chalk when you write.

If you can find the time for it, the following technique will be most helpful for the group of children in your class who have particular difficulty with blackboard reading. It will be of value even if you can devote no more than half an hour a week to it.

Start by having each child sit where he can see the blackboard clearly. Then write on the board groups of letters in *script,* classified according to height and other characteristics, and teach the child to analyze them. Thus:

1. Small letters: *a-c-e-i-o-u-m-n-r-s-u-v-w-x*
2. Closed letters: *a-e-o-s*
   a has a straight downstroke on the right
   e has a small loop
   o has a straight mark out to the right side, at the top
   s has a pointed top
3. Open letters: *c-m-n-r-u-v-w-x*
   c is the only one open on the right side
   m has three openings at the base
   n has two openings at the base
   r has one opening at the base
   u has one opening at the top, carries on from base
   v has one opening at the top, straight line top, right
   w has two openings at the top
   x is the only one with openings at the top, and at the base
   i is the only one of the short letters with a dot over it

4. Loop letters that go above the line: *b-f-h-k-l*
   b has an opening on the right top side
   f goes both high above the line, and below it
   h has an opening in the base
   k has an opening in the base, and a tuck in its side
   l is single loop tall letter
5. Loop letters that go below the line: *g-j-p-f-q-y-z*
   g is an *a*, with loop below the line
   j is the loop below, with a dot above the line
   p is loop with a bulb on the right
   q is an *o* with a loop to the right
   y has an open top with loop below
   z has an open left base, with loop below
6. *t* is tall, with a cross line

Complicated to begin with? Yes. But after you've taught the children to analyze the letters and after they have learned the letter forms so well that they can call out letters as you describe them verbally, you can work rapidly to improve their blackboard reading.

They have already ascertained how close they have to be to the blackboard to see it. Now each child moves back one seat so the writing will be just a little blurred and you put a list of related items on the board. For example:

Wild Animals

zebra	bear
tiger	giraffe
lion	hyena
boar	cougar
elephant	

Flowers

rose	daisy
aster	violet
nasturtium	peony
carnation	pink
trillium	

Toys

tops	electric trains
balls	cranes
kites	doll buggy
dolls	balloons
card games	bubble pipes

Other classifications that can be used include boys' names, girls' names, historical characters, rivers, states, countries.

Tell the children what the list includes and then ask them to read. Explain that the writing will be a little blurred but that, knowing what the words are, they can pick them out by identifying the forms of the letters. If a child reads "bear" for "boar," call his attention to the characteristics of the second letter until he recognizes the *o*. Teach him not to stare hard but to run his gaze from the beginning to the end of the word, back and forth, back and forth until he sees the form and identifies the letter by the form.

Now each child moves back another seat and you write another list on the board. Repeat the drill. The letters will be even hazier and it will take a little longer for the children to analyze the forms and identify the words. Keep their gaze shifting. Don't let them hunch forward in their seats, straining to see. Ask them to let the writing come to them. Encourage them to guess. If they're trying too hard, interrupt the drill for a moment to ease tension, then return to it.

Once the words have been read at this distance, each child now moves one seat forward again. Put another list on the board and then note what happens. Now at this distance, there will be much less blurring. The children will call the words more quickly and accurately.

In the next practice session, you can drill them at still greater distances. With each successful drill, their reading at the previous distance will improve.

You can do the same work with figures, dividing them into three categories: curved, straight, and curved-and-straight.

1. The curved are 3, 6, 8 and 0.
   3 has two openings to the left
   6 has one opening to the right and a curved base
   8 is closed at the top and the base
   0 is a complete curve
2. The straight figures are: 1, 7 and 4.
   1 is usually easy to see, except when it doubles and is 11
   4 is made of three straight lines
   7 is made of a straight line and a flat top
3. The curved-and-straight are: 2, 5 and 9.
   2 has a curve on the left, and a relatively flat base
   5 has a flat top, and a curve to the left
   9 has a closed, curved top, and a straight line

Once you begin to help children to understand and apply the principles of good vision, you will find yourself displaying great creativeness in developing your own effective methods and variations.

In their term papers, teachers who took my course on saving children's sight at a western university and, in the midst of it, began to apply the principles in their classrooms, presented many ideas they had tried successfully—usually quite simple ideas. Here are a few, just as they presented them in their papers. You may find them useful. They may suggest other ideas to you.

1. I move about a lot now while teaching so that the children will get the habit of shifting their gaze to watch me. When I introduced the long swing, the first grade loved it. Many children asked for it each day, even before I had a chance to announce that it would be a daily practice. We all found that it relieved eyestrain and relaxed tension.

2. We play a game each day in which all children with

glasses on take them off to clean them. And while glasses are off, they look at a letter on a card, shift to another letter on the same line, look at the first. They look, too, at a large letter, then at a smaller one a distance away. After a minute or two, all the letters seem clearer.

3. Each day the whole class does the palming. At first, it was not easy for the children. Some closed their eyes too tightly, but later on they got used to doing it. Immediately afterward, I have them look at the blackboard, or at a page of reading. They seem to see better.

4. Frequent use of blackboard, maps, pictures and even gestures, I find, keeps my pupils more interested and more relaxed. Whenever possible now, I refer to something outside, in the distance, to get a greater change of focus for the children.

5. I've found that well-planned assignments, involving shifting to board, map, books, etc., can do much to eliminate concentrated staring and provide frequent change of focus to relax the sight.

6. Some of my children had the habit of holding their books too near their faces. I have asked them to put a ruler between face and book. They enjoy doing this and often check up on themselves to see whether their book is still the required distance away. One little girl who held her book too close was already wearing glasses, and I took a special interest showing her how to do relaxation techniques and to increase her mobility. Now she can read without wearing her glasses, and when she claims her eyes feel strained, I let her palm for a few minutes. Her mother is very interested as she would much prefer her child not to have to wear glasses. I was gratified to know that the doctor told her that the child's eyes were getting stronger.

7. I have the children observe birds, airplanes, mountains, sky and trees. Sweeping the hand under pictures or words to emphasize left to right movement is very good.

8. I have them count objects such as beads, pegs and blocks for mobility and copy pictures or the alphabet from the blackboard for accommodation.

9. I ask the children to close their eyes and take imaginary trips. I also have them close their eyes and try to see an object I describe.

10. I use many action poems and songs such as "Go in and out the window," "Did you ever see a lassie?" and "Little Teapot," which necessitate pointing, swaying and bending.

11. During a walk, we count passers-by, umbrellas, cars, other things.

12. Every possible effort is being made to relieve strain in the classroom. The boardwork and seat work are varied so the children may rest their sight by looking far and near as much as possible during the day. I am using soft chalk so that it will be clearer. We rest frequently by looking around and standing for a stretch.

13. We remind one another when we are staring. Frequently, we palm for five minutes at a time. Some of the children will palm, without being told to do so, when they are waiting for others to put wraps away.

14. The benefits derived from blinking have been explained to the children. We remind one another about it. We practice flashing or quick sight in our word drills. I admit that, before taking this course, I was frequently guilty of telling my poor readers to "look hard" at a word, when I should have let them only flash back and forth easily.

15. We play games of feeling things with our eyes shut and guessing what they are.

16. We listen to phonograph records while palming.

17. We are fifty in number in our room, and the overcrowding and noise make for strain. That is one reason why I find so much relief in having the children palm and do the long swing.

18. I am watching the reading distance of the pupils. Some have a habit of resting their books on the waistline while reading. They are constantly hearing, "Hold your book up."

19. We use games such as "Simon Says," act out songs, finger plays and breathing drills. It is up to the teacher to make these drills profitable to the sight. For instance, in playing "Simon Says," instead of moving just the thumbs up and down, the whole body can be moved, pointing to north, south, east and west.

20. Many games and drills can be used in arithmetic to aid in getting the children to shift their gaze. In one such drill, I put two sets of identical problems on the board, then have two children (from opposite sides) work them, writing answers as quickly as possible. The other children keep looking from one contestant to the other to see who is ahead.

21. In reading, I have the children look in their books to find phrases I've written on the board, thus getting near to far shifting.

22. Instead of passing out as many dittoed sheets as I did in the past, I now put at least part of the assignment on the board for children to copy. In this way, they must shift their gaze from near to far.

23. I call on pupils sitting in different parts of the room so the others will turn and shift.

24. I point to different objects in the room as illustrations while explaining something.

Helping children to preserve and strengthen their sight is rewarding work. You will be pioneering in an area that has been greatly neglected, making a constructive contribution toward replacing do-nothingism and even downright defeatism.

You will neither be offering nor advocating a panacea. Inculcating good habits of seeing is not a substitute for medical care when it's needed. You will not be diagnosing or prescribing for eye diseases—only teaching children how to make best use of their vision.

You'll be rewarded by noteworthy improvement in many children whose eyesight has begun to fail and by the knowledge that, in the others as well, you are helping to develop good habits of seeing that will be important to them all their lives.

And if the experience of other teachers counts, you can expect an improvement in the scholastic achievements of your students and, not least of all, a more pleasant, relaxed classroom.

Chapter XXII

Recording Your Progress

You are about to start working to rebuild your sight. The final reward, the ultimate improvement, will come some months from now. But there will be rewards on the way, too, as you measure your progress.

Much of the work you will be doing lends itself to such measurement. From day to day and week to week, you will

SAMPLE PROGRESS REPORT (NEARSIGHT)

Date started: Jan. 10th

	I						II							
	M	T	W	T	F	S	S	M	T	W	T	F	S	S
Time spent without glasses, (total hours)	1¼	1¼	2	2	2½	4	5½	2	2½	2½	2	2½	4½	6
Sunning (times a day)	3	3	4	4	3	5	6	4	4	3	4	4	5	4
Palming (times a day)	3	3	4	4	3	5	6	4	4	3	4	4	5	4
Long Swing	✓	✓	✓	✓	✓	✓	✓	✓	✓	✓	✓	✓	✓	✓
Movie			✓						✓					
Letter Board I, both eyes (distance)	2'2"	2'5"		2'7"	3'	3'4"								
Cord fusion	✓	✓	✓	✓	✓	✓	✓	✓	✓	✓	✓	✓	✓	✓
Domino drill								✓	✓		✓	✓	✓	✓
Playing card drill, both eyes								✓	✓		✓	✓	✓	✓
Letter Board II, both eyes														

Your list should include the following drills: short swings, counting objects and colors, edging objects, vertical shifting, games, alternate sunning and palming, ruler shifting, tossing ball. Letter Board 1 (each eye), dice throwing, Gettysburg Address, ring fusion, solitaire, domino wheel (each eye), watch to clock, ring fusion to letter board I, solitaire (each eye), lights in mirror, ring fusion on jumbled numbers, perforated board sunning, yardstick

Fig. 37 Practice Record

be able to go without glasses for progressively longer periods. If you are working to improve your distance vision, you'll be able to note progress in the gradually increasing distances at which you can do the cord fusion and the letter board, jumbled numbers, playing card and other accommodation drills. If you are working to improve your close point vision, you'll be able to measure your improvement in the shorter and shorter distances at which you are able to do the drills, and also in your ability to read smaller and smaller print.

Measuring your progress is important. The more you're aware of improvement, the more you will be stimulated to keep working forward. Your confidence will increase, too, and confidence, in itself, seems to be an important psychological factor in building sight.

In addition, it is also helpful to keep a practice record such as shown in Fig. 37. The sample is for nearsightedness, but similar records can be kept for other vision problems.

III							IV							V						
M	T	W	T	F	S	S	M	T	W	T	F	S	S	M	T	W	T	F	S	S
3/4/4	2½/3/4	2½/4/5	2½/4/4	2/5/4	6/6/6	7/7/6	3/4/4	3/4/5	3/5/6	2½/4/3	3/4/4	6/5/5	6/6/6	3/4/4	3½/4/4	3½/5/5	3/4/5	3/4/5	7/6/6	7/6/6
✓	✓	✓ ✓	✓	✓	✓	✓ ✓	✓	✓	✓	✓	✓	✓	✓	✓	✓ ✓	✓	✓	✓	✓	✓
							4'	4'6"			4'9"	5'3"	5'8"							
✓	✓	✓	✓	✓	✓	✓	✓	✓	✓	✓	✓	✓	✓	✓	✓	✓	✓	✓	✓	✓
													2'4"	2'7"			3'	3'4"	3'8"	4'2"

fusion, reading (each eye), Letter board I (each eye), jumbled numbers (both eyes), channel yardstick to domino wheel, playing card drill (each eye), near to far on magazine ads, red shifter in distance, jumbled numbers (each eye), plate fusion, channel yardstick to letter board I, reading (both eyes), ring fusion to jumbled letters, toss cards, letter board II (each eye), jumbled letters (both eyes), and card fusion with yardstick.

Fig. 37 Continued

You'll need only a few pages of graph paper—or you can rule off ordinary white paper. Across the top of a page write in the dates. You can join several sheets together with cellophane tape to provide enough columns for the twelve-week program and for additional work as well.

In the left-hand column, list first all the drills which are to be done daily throughout the program. Then, list the other drills which vary from week to week.

Each day, as you do the work called for, check it off in the proper square.

You can also note on your practice record the time spent each day without glasses, the starting distances for accommodation and other drills and the number of the graduated print you're able to read without glasses when you begin, then note distances at which you can work and the numbers of graduated print you can read as you go along.

The practice record will help in several ways.

With it, of course, you can make certain that you are doing all the work called for.

It will also enable you to make substitutions now and then that can help your progress. Boredom in practice is not desirable. Wherever possible, a variety of drills has been provided and there are changes from week to week to help avoid boredom. Suppose, however, that on a day when your program calls for domino wheel practice, you feel just a little tired of that drill. A glance at your record may show that you haven't had to use another accommodation drill— perhaps, jumbled numbers—recently, and you can substitute it for the domino wheel drill that day.

Finally, keeping a practice record often provides a psychological lift. Many students have reported that it adds to their feeling of accomplishment when they check off each day's work.

Index